Sunrise over Pangnirtung
The Story of Otto Schaefer, M.D.

Gerald W. Hankins, M.D.

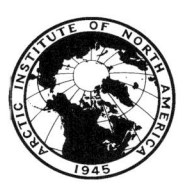

Komatik Series, Number 6
The Arctic Institute of North America
of the University of Calgary

© 2000 The Arctic Institute of North America and Gerald Hankins

All rights reserved. No part of this publication may be reproduced, stored in a retrieval system or transmitted in any form or by any means, electronic, mechanical, photocopying, recording or otherwise (except brief passages for purposes of review), without the prior permission of the copyright holders.

Published by The Arctic Institute of North America
of the University of Calgary
2500 University Drive N.W.
Calgary, Alberta, Canada   T2N 1N4

Canadian Cataloguing in Publication Data

Hankins, Gerald W.
      Sunrise over Pangnirtung

   (Komatik series, ISSN 0840-4488 ; 6)
   Includes bibliographical references and index.
   ISBN 0-919034-97-7

      1. Schaefer, Otto, 1919- 2. Physicians—Canada, Northern—Biography. 3. Medical care—Canada, Northern. I. Arctic Institute of North America. II. Title. III. Series.
R464.S39H36 2000   610'.92   C00-910723-1

Credits:
Copyediting by Luisa Alexander Izzo
Indexing by Judy Dunlop, Edmonton, Alberta
Cartography by Marilyn Croot, Sun Mountain Graphics, Calgary, Alberta
Interior and cover design by Jeremy Drought, Last Impression Publishing
      Service, Calgary, Alberta
Cover photo of Pangnirtung, Baffin Island, Nunavut, October 1999,
      by Jerry Kobalenko
Printed and bound by Houghton Boston, Saskatoon, Saskatchewan

PRINTED IN CANADA

*Nowhere has knowledge been purchased
at greater cost of privation and suffering.*

FRIDTJOF NANSEN

Table of Contents

- Foreword vii
- Preface ix
- Acknowledgements xi
- A Map of the Canadian Arctic xiii

1 • Crisis in Cumberland Sound 1
2 • Life under the Nazis 7
3 • A New Canadian 12
4 • Into the Depths of the Arctic 19
5 • Early Days at Aklavik 23
6 • Witness for the Prosecution 31
7 • Patients and Characters 36
8 • Didi and the Arctic 44
9 • Shamans and Missionaries 48
10 • The Final Months at Aklavik 52
11 • On Board the *C.D. Howe* 56
12 • The Icy Waters of the Eastern Arctic 62
13 • Baffin Island 67
14 • Early Days in Pangnirtung 74
15 • Etuangat 79
16 • The Hard Life 83
17 • Folk Lore and Ingenuity 87
18 • Darkness and Light 91
19 • Challenges 96
20 • Travels by Dog Team 100
21 • White-Knuckle Moments 105
22 • Allies, Most of the Time 109
23 • Hunting and Survival 115
24 • "The Arctic We Knew" 123

25 • The Turning Point 127
26 • The Yukon 133
27 • On the Launching Pad 138
28 • The Changing North 141
29 • Surveys Across the North 144
30 • The Executioners 150
31 • Human Adaptation 157
32 • Nutrition and Malnutrition 162
33 • A Changing and Crumbling Society 169
34 • Circumpolar Medical Conference 173
35 • At the Heart of Controversy 179
36 • Native Women's Conference 182
37 • Didi 185
38 • Guest Lecturer 190
39 • Honoured by the North 193
40 • Papers and Publications 196
41 • Full Circle 199
42 • Cruel Blows 204
43 • Etuangat Elevated 208
44 • Living Memories 212
45 • If Otto Schaefer hadn't gone to the Arctic 219

- Appendix: Selected Papers of Otto Schaefer 223
- References 234
- Index 239

Foreword

As is often the case with people of prominence, Dr. Otto Schaefer's reputation preceded by some years our eventual meeting. I first heard about him in 1961, when I was medical officer of the Eastern Arctic Patrol aboard the *C.D. Howe*, a government icebreaker that each year was converted into a hospital ship. Its itinerary included visits to some 25 Inuit settlements in the Eastern Arctic. One of these was Pangnirtung, where Dr. Schaefer had been the resident medical officer for two years in the mid-1950s. While the *C.D. Howe* docked there for two days, I learned a little about Otto from the nursing staff of the Anglican hospital and, through an interpreter, from the local Inuit people. Although the accounts of Otto's medical achievements were impressive, my greatest surprise was the eclectic spread of his other interests and pursuits. These included aboriginal archaeology, traditional Inuit medicine (with an emphasis on shamanistic beliefs), and his study of the local Inuit language.

Soon after completing the medical patrol, I was posted to Iqaluit on Baffin Island for two years, then transferred to Edmonton. It was there that I finally met Otto! My first reaction was amazement at his energy and unrestrained enthusiasm for life. Otto never walked: he only ran. It was as if, in his formative years, he had skipped that middle step between crawling and running.

In Edmonton, my family became close friends with the Schaefers, and Otto and I became close medical colleagues. At that time, the North was opening up. World War II had brought about the construction of airports across the North. More sophisticated safety installations were established, road transportation was improved, and the United States established the gigantic Distant Early Warning system (the DEW Line) to prevent air attacks from Russia. Finally, the government of the day declared a "Vision of the North," which would provide significant resources for expansion of health services.

It was always an adventure to go north, but to go with Otto was a command performance. During a typical visit, after we completed our clinical routine, Otto commenced house calls, partly in search of recalcitrants who did not attend clinics, and partly to pursue his special studies relating to nutrition, myopia, diabetes, and foetal alcohol syndrome. One of his expressions was: "We must always keep an open and inquiring mind."

Eventually our geographical proximity was to end. Otto took leave to pursue studies leading to his specialist degree in internal medicine, and I left for Toronto. In 1973, I came to Ottawa where, after three years as principal medical officer, I became director general of Indian/Inuit Health.

Otto never did decelerate. A plethora of research papers emanated from his office at the Charles Camsell Hospital in Edmonton. His numerous awards will be fully detailed in this book. He is a disciplined and dutiful man. God bless the Otto Schaefers of this planet. There are not many of them, and we do need them so very much.

Brian Brett, M.D.
Former Director General
Indian and Inuit Health
Department of National Health and Welfare

Preface

Dr. Otto Schaefer, an outstanding medical doctor who gave 32 years of his life to caring for the Inuit, pioneered health care for those living in the barren lands. Growing up during the Nazi regime in Germany, he came to Canada in 1951 and spent time at Edmonton's Royal Alexandra and Charles Camsell hospitals. In 1953 he was posted to Aklavik in the Mackenzie Delta. Later he spent two years in Pangnirtung on Baffin Island ("paradise on earth," he calls it) and another two years in Whitehorse, Yukon Territory.

He learned the Inuktitut language, lived in igloos while visiting remote Inuit camps, removed retained placentas by the light of a seal oil lamp, ate raw frozen caribou meat, and travelled by dog team—sometimes through blinding blizzards. His friendship and rapport with the Inuit enabled him to travel from Old Crow to Cape Dyer, treating sick people and collecting details about their health problems for the Northern Medical Research Unit. His contribution to the medical literature was astounding: more than 100 papers and publications, in addition to contributions to textbooks.

Otto Schaefer has received widespread recognition with honours, awards, tributes and medals from several universities, governments, and other institutions. Retired since 1985, he now lives in Edmonton, where his home is filled with Inuit carvings, caribou horns and polar bear skins. But his heart—and his thoughts—remain in the Arctic.

I first met Otto Schaefer in 1994. A medical colleague who was familiar with my two previous biographies and had worked in the Yukon with Otto was adamant: "You simply must talk to him." I followed his advice, but Otto was not in favour of the idea. Later, perhaps under some pressure, he relented.

It has been a privilege for me to write the life story of a man who loved the Inuit. As their friend, he rejoiced in some ways and agonized in others as outside forces changed their way of life forever. His story spans the period of rapid transition from the dog team and sealskin tent of yesteryear to today's snowmobile and oil-heated frame house.

While acknowledging the magnitude of Otto Schaefer's contribution to health care in the North, it has been my intention right from the outset to avoid writing an erudite book replete with medical jargon. But I have attempted to ensure that most statements are verifiable. My sincere hope is that this book will appeal to all kinds of readers.

I readily admit that much of the book is written from the perspective of Otto Schaefer: interviews with Otto and his publications, diaries (1953–57), and letters were my chief sources. But much help came too from books, newspaper clippings, letters, and talks with a great number of colleagues, associates, family members, and former government employees. I am fortunate to have had access to so much fine material. My own experience serving as a medical doctor in the Inuvik Regional Hospital, Northwest Territories, should lend some authenticity to the record. The photographs, unless otherwise stated, are from the collection of Otto Schaefer.

The word "Eskimo" remains entrenched in the minds of many people, but in this book I will call Canada's northernmost population by the name they use: "Inuit" (the people).

Why "Sunrise over Pangnirtung"? I think it fair to say that the work of Otto Schaefer helped to bring the dawn of a new day for the health care of Northerners. "Pangnirtung" I chose because the treeless fjords and cliffs of this hamlet on Baffin Island were a paradise on earth for Otto Schaefer and his late wife, Editha.

Acknowledgements

Anyone undertaking the job of writing the life story of a distinguished person is well aware of the need to rely upon the help of a host of other persons. This author has received such help in abundance—and is grateful.

Dr. Otto Schaefer, the central figure of this book, proved to be a most willing subject during the delightful hours we talked together. He went to great pains to access obscure details for me and made available for my use quantities of files, clippings, medical journals, and diaries. There can be few people more conscientious and supremely honest than Otto. Further, most of the pictures in this book were taken by his discerning camera. I recognized early on that these pictures were treasures. I remain grateful to Otto for the use of these pictures and to those people who gave me permission to use pictures from other publications.

I owe a debt of gratitude to Dr. David and Mrs. Joan Boon of Kamloops, who first told me about Otto's distinguished career among the Inuit. I am also indebted to Theresa White of Kelowna, the first person to read and critique the manuscript and pronounce it "a good story."

Helpful personal communications have come from Gerry and Betty Amerongen, Dr. Maurice and Mrs. Renata Beare, Dr. Lyell Black, Dr. David Boon, Dr. Brian Brett, Kay Dier, Shirley Donaghue, Dr. Buzz Edwards, Jack Grainge, Emmi Nemetz, Winnie Paege, Dr. Dick Rossall, Iris Stout, Elva Taylor, Norma Westgate, Taoya White, and others.

I appreciated the critiquing of the manuscript by Dr. C.S. Houston and Dr. R.G. Williamson of the University of Saskatchewan.

A timely and much-appreciated grant from the Alberta Medical Foundation allowed the final editing and publishing to proceed.

Lastly, I have valued the patience and diligence of Dr. Karen McCullough, Editor for the Arctic Institute of North America. A strong proponent of precision and clarity, Karen made me think twice about sources and references and thereby did much to improve the overall quality of the book. Luisa Izzo, the copy editor, rightfully questioned many of my fuzzy declarations.

My wife Alison has shown great patience and tolerance of my writing endeavours. I am grateful not only for her understanding, but also for her encouragement along the way.

I may have unintentionally forgotten to mention others who assisted me with this wonderful task. Please forgive me for doing so.

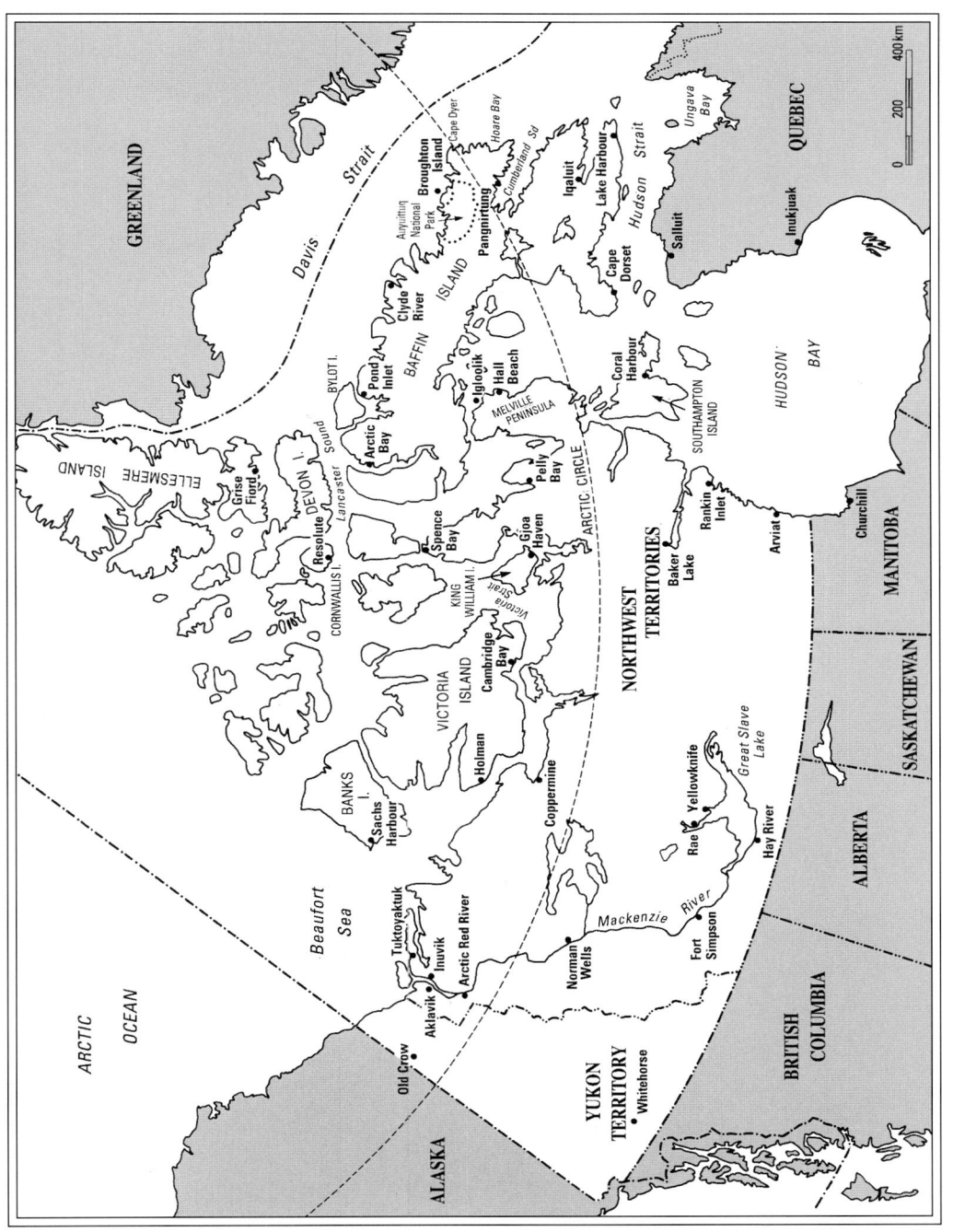

1
Crisis in Cumberland Sound

THE dogs seemed to know it was a matter of life and death. Breath steaming from flared nostrils, tails pointing straight back and hind legs straining, they sprinted through the Arctic darkness over the sea ice of Cumberland Sound.

Auk, Auk! Ai, Ai! (Left, right!) Etuangat, seated on the grub box at the front of the *komatik* (sled), urged them on. No need to use his long whip. Once again, spurred into action by an emergency call that had reached the little mission hospital at Pangnirtung well after midnight, the hospital's dog team was serving as Baffin Island's ambulance. In desperate search of medical help, an Inuit driver and his panting dogs had raced some 80 km from the camp at Illongaya, near the northern end of the Sound. A young woman, bleeding heavily, had fallen unconscious and appeared near death, he said. She would never survive the rough trip by dog sled.

Dr. Otto Schaefer, resident physician at Pangnirtung, hopped out of his warm bed. Since his arrival in the fall of 1955, he had made a few trips by dog team to Inuit camps around Cumberland Sound and over the mountains to places like Broughton Island on Davis Strait. But "house calls" for emergencies like this were another matter. He pulled on long underwear, a woolen shirt, and pants and over these his outer caribou pants and parka. He wore *kamiks* (boots) of caribou hide, an inner pair with hair against his skin and an outer pair with hair to the outside; over these he pulled on slippers of polar bear skin. He knew that in March an Arctic blizzard could strike at any time without warning.

His Inuit helper, Etuangat Aksayook, though 20 years older, seemed to move a lot faster. While Otto rummaged around in the hospital for the emergency box, a good supply of antibiotics, and equipment to cross-match blood and give transfusions, Etuangat rounded up the dogs, each nestled deep in the snow, and harnessed them up. Then he found a place for the tired man from Illongaya to rest.

After six months as Medical Officer for the Eastern Arctic at Pang (as they called it), Otto had developed a healthy respect for the North. "You don't play games with one of the most harsh and unforgiving climates on earth," he said. Emergency or not, he and Etuangat carefully loaded food, a tent, sleeping bags, and medical supplies into boxes on the *komatik*, lashed the boxes securely with strips of tough hide, and covered all with caribou and polar bear skins.

By 3:00 a.m., the seven leaping, yelping dogs were all harnessed up in fan-shaped formation, tied by lines of varying length to the main rope pulling the sled. Otto appreciated the need for the fan-shaped configuration to adapt to Baffin's rough, rocky tundra and jagged tidal ice (the result of the ebb and flow of the tide during freeze-up), but it did mean stopping to get off the sled and untangle lines now and then.

Then they were off into the inky blackness of an Arctic night. First they had to cross the no-man's-land of tidal ice—the hardest part of the journey—to get onto the smooth, snow-covered sea ice. The dogs needed no urging; in fact, they had to be restrained for fear the sled would overturn or smash against the sharp mounds and pillars of ice. On the smooth sea ice, Etuangat needed only to shout commands to keep them on course as they raced ahead.

Somehow he knew where to go, even with nothing to go by but the stars and an uncanny sense of direction. Hired several years before as doctor's helper and interpreter, this wise, middle-aged Inuk had taught Otto many things during his six months at Pang. What's more, Etuangat had learned a bit about medicine and more than once had got Otto out of trouble. As the new doctor on the scene, Otto had once found himself perplexed by the case of another young woman, whose condition had defied diagnosis. Etuangat suggested that she might have nothing physically wrong with her, but simply be neurotic. "She acts up like this for every new doctor," he said. Otto later found out that this diagnosis was right on target.

Etuangat, called "Wanga" by Otto's young son Lothar, understood English well enough, but annoyed Otto at first by making a point of answering his questions in Inuktitut. In reply to Otto's question about an urgent matter, he answered, "I'll speak English when I go to your country; you speak Inuktitut when you come to mine." Those were his last words to Otto in English. Otto had only a smattering of the Inuit language; from then on, he forged ahead to learn it. In time it would open many doors for him.

Sitting on the warm polar bear hide covering the boxes, Otto began to shiver. A bitter crosswind howling across the Sound swirled a drift of fine snow around the moving sled. He wanted to hop off and run with the dogs, as he often did, but they were travelling too fast, and he didn't want to lose any time. The cold was one thing; the searing, biting wind, another. He had heard of people being trapped in a blizzard, lost in the gale of a raging snowstorm where they could not even see their own feet.

The moment Otto was waiting for suddenly arrived: two dogs got tangled in their traces and fell together, a writhing mass in the snow. While Etuangat disentangled them, Otto jumped off the sled and tried a few calisthenics in his bulky clothing. Since the dogs were slowing down, he decided to run alongside. He soon warmed up.

A lean, bouncy 37-year-old of below-average height, he hardly looked the type to revel in hardships and tough conditions. Emigrating from Germany to Canada in 1951, he had worked first as a hired labourer on his uncle's farm in Saskatchewan, then as a junior intern in a hospital, a lowly job compared with his status as a consultant specialist in internal medicine in Germany. No sooner had he passed the Canadian qualifying exams in medicine than he asked to be posted to the Arctic by the Department of National Health and Welfare. After two years at Aklavik in the delta of the great Mackenzie River, he had been sent to Baffin Island.

Back in 1616, the British navigator-explorer William Baffin had explored the coasts of Canada's largest island and written: "A dark and angry sea, a lifeless rocky coast, ice and a freezing wind" (Mountfield,

1974:44). Yet after six months, Otto Schaefer was captivated by the place. And so was his wife Editha (Didi), who had come from Germany in 1952 to join him, knowing she would be facing the rigours of the Arctic with her adventurous husband.

Just a hint of dawn lit the velvety, black northern sky when the rescue team neared its destination. They could see nothing, but the howling and yelping of distant dogs announced they were close. It was comforting to know they were near, although the welcome sounds would soon change into snarls with the fights and scraps that are inevitable when one group of dogs invades another's territory.

Alerted by the dogs, several people came to greet the two men from the hospital. They took them to a small sealskin winter tent filled with people. No one spoke: only the whimpering of a newborn baby broke the silence. The light of a dim seal-oil lamp revealed a young, desperately ill Inuit woman lying off to one side and moaning softly. Otto knelt beside her and flicked on his flashlight. Her eyes were sunken, her face ashen, and her breathing shallow and irregular. He felt her forehead—cool and clammy; her pulse—weak and thready. Her undergarments were soaked with blood.

She had lost a lot of blood and it needed to be replaced. Here's where Otto would put heavy reliance on his sturdy helper: "Etuangat, she needs a blood transfusion. I need to test the blood of several of these young fellows and if I find blood that is compatible with hers, I'd like to take half a litre from two of them. Tell them it's essential that we do this to save her life," he said. In a soft but firm voice, Etuangat explained the instructions. One man pursed his lips, and another nodded his head slightly, but no one said anything.

After emptying the small tent of everyone but the patient's husband, Otto got down on his knees and inserted the packing he hoped would control the bleeding. With a syringe and needle, he took a small quantity of blood from her arm for cross-matching. It was backbreaking work, and even on his knees, he felt his head brush against the roof of the tent.

Two of the "volunteers" had blood that was compatible with that of the patient. Otto brought them into the tent, collected blood from them in a sterile transfusion bottle, and proceeded to give her slowly a litre of blood. She needed far more, but this was a start. By the time they had finished and were ready to lie down in their sleeping bags for a short rest, daylight had come.

There was no time to waste. After a cup of hot tea and a good chew on a half-frozen joint of raw caribou, they prepared to go back. They bundled their patient into Otto's sleeping bag, added several caribou skins, and tied her securely to the top of the *komatik*. The wind had died down and, apart from the bumps and jolts travelling over the tidal ice, it was a smooth trip back to Pangnirtung. In the hospital, Otto gave his patient more blood and then operated to remove retained fragments of placenta. It was hardly major surgery; in fact, it could even be called routine. Otto made little of it.

When he spoke to the young woman before she left for home a few days later, it was to give her advice for the care of her baby and for

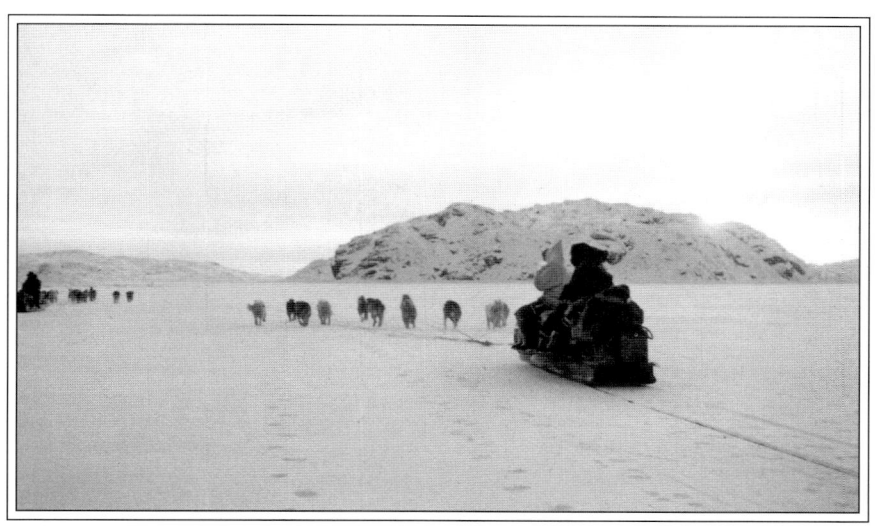

Otto Schaefer's first long dog team trip to visit Inuit campsites in Cumberland Sound, February 1956. Otto's sled, with Etuangat and his son Amosie, is in the foreground. The travellers are near Illongaya (called "Bonne Accord" by the whalers and on official maps), about 70 km west of Pangnirtung.

herself during her next pregnancy. Had he and Etuangat not raced their dogs through the darkness to Illongaya camp, the young Inuit woman would almost certainly have died. Yet Otto might have forgotten the incident completely, had it not been for the disabling backache that crippled him for days afterward.

In later years, however, he would write a brief account of this nocturnal dash across the ice of Cumberland Sound for a medical journal, as an example of "some of the difficult circumstances still prevailing in wide parts of the Eastern Arctic" (Schaefer, 1959:249).

2
Life under the Nazis

EVEN as a boy of eight in far-off Germany, Otto Schaefer had burned with a passion for the Canadian Arctic. The Land of the Midnight Sun, with its icebergs, tundra, polar bears, seals, blizzards, sundogs and northern lights, captured his heart and overflowed into his dreams and reveries. Someday he would go and see it all for himself, he said. Even more, he would live and work with the hardy and heroic Eskimos.

A book from his older brother, Joseph, had sparked his young imagination. Written by Greenlandic-Danish Knud Rasmussen, it was entitled *Groenlaendische Sagen* (Tales of Greenland). The book's folklore, myths, tales, and legends captivated him. Three years later, Joseph gave him another book, which would set the course of his life. Actually it was a set of two volumes written by Franz Boas, bearing the titles *The Central Eskimo* (Boas, 1888) and *Baffin-Land* (Boas, 1885).

Boas had gone to Cumberland Sound in June 1883 on the *Germania*. The German Polar Commission ship was returning to evacuate the International Polar Year team from the German Polar Station. A young geographer and ethnographer, Boas was planning a year of fieldwork to study various aspects of Inuit culture and society and their relation to the arctic environment. In preparation, he had began to learn Inuktitut, studied British Admiralty charts, and learned techniques of topography and cartography. His detailed topographic surveys and documentation of traditional Inuit place names would become a major contribution: he produced the first map of this area based on precise geodetic measurements (Müller-Wille, 1998).

But Boas made his greatest contribution by publishing *The Central Eskimo*, which remains a classic of Inuit anthropology more than a century later. A pioneer anthropologist, Boas went on to become a curator at the Museum of Natural History in New York and founded the first anthropology department in North America, at Clark University in Worcester, Massachusetts.

Besides mapping, Boas was requested by his government to look for iron ore—and not to repeat Martin Frobisher's fiasco of 300 years earlier. After returning to England in 1576 with chunks of ore from Baffin Island, Frobisher got the startling news that they contained gold. Sailing back to Baffin in 1577 and 1578, Frobisher excavated almost 1500 tons of the supposed gold ore. Unfortunately, his "precious ore" proved to be worthless iron pyrites: fool's gold (Kenyon, 1975).

Joseph had seen his young brother poring over maps hour after hour and figured he could not go wrong with this kind of a gift. The book fired the imagination of eleven-year-old Otto Schaefer; then and there he set his mind on going to Baffin Island, in particular to Cumberland Sound. He would have to wait many years, overcome many obstacles, and endure devastating tragedies—including the destruction of his country—before he could see for himself the bays and mountains of Baffin Island. But he would stay on course.

Otto was born on October 2, 1919 in the Schaefer family home in Betzdorf, a small town located 23 km east of Bonn on a tributary of the Rhine. At that time Bonn, birthplace of the great Beethoven and capital of West Germany from 1949 to 1990, was a university city of about 100,000. Otto's start in life was hardly auspicious. Being the fourth in a line of boys certainly did not confer any special privileges. And from a year and a half after his birth, when a much-wanted girl was born, Otto existed in the shadow of lovable Lizbeth with the golden curls.

What's more, his mother worried that he was retarded. Her anxiety intensified when Lizbeth actually began speaking before he did. Greatly concerned, she took him to their family physician just before his third birthday. The doctor examined him, but found nothing amiss. Then he pronounced: "I can't find anything wrong with him apart from bone-laziness. Unless I miss my guess, he'll soon start talking—and once he gets going, he'll never stop." His prognosis was not far wrong.

Otto's teenage years in Germany were a time of ferment and tyranny as the burgeoning Nazi party seized control and crushed all opposition. Otto's father, a senior administrator with the national railway, found himself blacklisted and demoted because "only politically reliable people could be trusted with that kind of important job." Otto got into trouble too: his refusal to join the Hitler Youth put him under suspicion. He also refused to join the Nazi-inspired mass movement against Jews. It bothered him to see Jewish people subjected to verbal insults, spitting, and destruction of their homes and shops. At school his sneering teacher called him "Jew lover" and made him sit alone on a bench, but he just couldn't keep silent while the underdogs suffered. He readily admits it was scary at the time, but it stiffened his backbone and set a lifelong trend—a stubborn willingness to take an unpopular stance. If some idea or cause was worthy of support or criticism, he would not hesitate to say so, even if it meant ridicule and scorn.

Contrary to his mother's fears, Otto excelled at school. He majored in the humanities, studying Greek and Latin along with some French and English, the latter as an elective. At the age of 14, he decided he wanted to be a medical doctor. Later he was to say, "I was always interested in biology, and medicine would permit me to put my knowledge to practical use." And of course the people of the Canadian North were still in the forefront of his thinking. In his planning, he had failed to take into account the Nazi spy system. One of his own high school classmates betrayed him. Police and party officials searched his home and confiscated "seditious material," including booklets on the outlawed Scout movement. Attempting to register in the Faculty of Medicine at Bonn University, he was told to "get right with the Party first."

Later a friend, a nominal Nazi, told Otto that if he volunteered to serve with the infantry for a couple of years, he would then be considered "patriotic enough" to register at the university. It was 1938, a year with war clouds on the horizon. Somehow, in spite of his poor eyesight (astigmatism and myopia), he passed the medical and joined the infantry. Had he stayed in the infantry, he almost certainly would have been killed. Only three men from his regiment would survive the war; all the rest would lose their lives in the fighting on the Russian front after the 1941 invasion.

As it was, when war broke out in 1939, Otto and others were encouraged to get on with their studies in medicine to meet the need for medical officers in the Wehrmacht (German army). During these university years, his class studied for six or seven months in uniform at the University of Bonn and spent the rest of each year on active service at one of the battle fronts.

In the large army hospital at Sevastopol in the Crimea, he worked as a doctor's assistant, helping with operations on wounded soldiers. During the Battle of the Bulge, near the end of the war, he got his fill of seeing young men's bodies shattered by bombs and bullets. He wanted to be loyal to his country, though he hated the Nazis and regretted having to be on their side. "But in war," he said, "you have no choice, no matter what your ideology. If you do something against the war effort and are discovered, you know you will be shot."

In 1944, Otto graduated in Medicine from the University of Heidelberg. He then wrote a dissertation, which allowed him to qualify in medicine and call himself Doctor Medicinae. Professor Richard Siedbach, one of the senior men reviewing students' dissertations, gave him the highest possible mark. Otto again served on the front lines, now a medical officer in the retreating German Army, as the death knell sounded for the once-mighty Third Reich. He was captured in Upper Bavaria just before his country surrendered in May 1945 and remained behind barbed wire until July.

He returned to find his home town of Betzdorf destroyed and his parents' home bombed into rubble. Incendiary bombs had destroyed precious books and all their family pictures, including those of Otto as a child. His country was in ruins, and Adolf Hitler lay dead by his own hand.

For the next year Otto's work as an intern in surgery, obstetrics, and pediatrics in a Heidelberg hospital gave him good general experience, but he really wanted training in the specialty of internal medicine. In

January 1946, the same Professor Siedbach welcomed Otto back to the University of Heidelberg, where he obtained his specialist degree in 1950. Then followed a year as assistant to the head of the Department of Internal Medicine at Baden-Baden's city hospital before he left his home country for Canada.

During the long years of violence and barbarism, Otto sometimes despaired, but he never gave up hope of realizing his childhood dream. Somehow, in the midst of bombs, machine-gun fire, and exploding rockets, his vision of the Inuit living in the windswept Arctic snows spoke to him of peace. Now the door to that dream was opening.

3

A New Canadian

ON July 1, 1951, the S.S. *Atlantic* docked in Halifax harbour. Two minutes after the gangplank hit the wet asphalt of the wharf, Otto Schaefer was hurrying down it to set foot on the ground of his newly adopted country. He wished for nothing more than to head north to Baffin Island and start working. Sadly, "a whole tank trap of obstacles" (as he called them) blocked his way.

Before leaving Germany, he had told Canadian immigration authorities of his offer to work as a physician for Indian and Eskimo Health Services in the Eastern Arctic. At that time, however, Canada wanted special categories of immigrants, such as agricultural workers and miners. True, doctors were needed in the North, but the Department of Immigration had its policy. To further complicate matters, Otto would have to find a Canadian sponsor to become a landed immigrant. Bill Schneider, an uncle-in-law from Goodsoil in northern Saskatchewan, agreed to sponsor him. He offered Otto a job as an "agricultural worker" and even sent him a cheque in case Immigration wanted confirmation.

Passing through Ottawa on the long train journey to Saskatchewan, Otto stopped to make enquiries at Indian and Eskimo Health Services. Officials advised him to go to the Charles Camsell Hospital in Edmonton, a referral centre for Native people from the western provinces and the Yukon and Northwest Territories. But as an immigrant doctor from central Europe, Otto would have to pass exams like other foreign graduates. His considerable experience and specialty degree in internal medicine would not exempt him.

It was like hiring a skilled carpenter to extract rusty nails from a pile of old lumber, but Otto didn't mind. He chopped wood and forked hay for his uncle, who did his best to help him settle down in the new country. Being in a German-speaking community helped Otto to overcome his homesickness.

At the first opportunity, Otto travelled to Saskatoon to find out what the provincial College of Physicians and Surgeons would require of him. First, he would have to pass exams in the basic medical sciences to get an "enabling certificate." Then he could apply for a job as junior intern in a hospital, repeating what he had done five years before. A couple of months after arrival, he took work as an orderly at the provincial (mental) hospital in North Battleford. Studying on the job, he passed the exams in basic sciences. In October, he began looking for a Saskatchewan hospital in need of junior interns; but all four teaching hospitals had their full complement.

Hoping for a vacancy at the Royal Alexandra Hospital in Edmonton was a long shot, but Otto thought it worth a try. At that time the Royal Alex was the largest hospital in western Canada for surgical emergencies and obstetrics; it would be the ideal place to gain the experience he

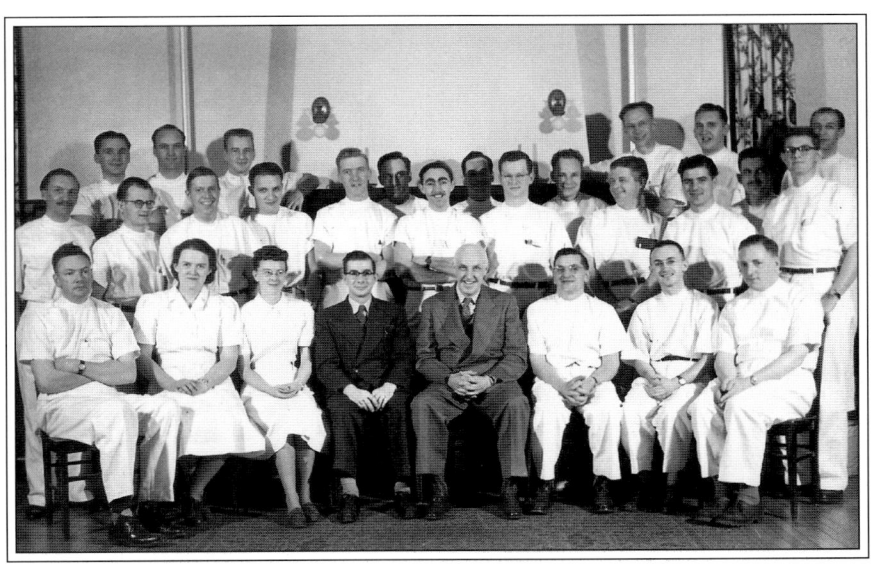

Interns and residents at the Royal Alexandra Hospital, Edmonton, in 1952. Otto Schaefer is the second from the left in the middle row.

wanted before going to the isolated North. And it would be a great advantage to be in the same city as the Charles Camsell Hospital, which he visualized as the jumping-off place for the Arctic. To his great delight, the Royal Alex accepted him, and on November 1, 1951 he put on a white uniform and took up his duties along with recent medical graduates and a few other foreign doctors.

But yet another obstacle barred his path: Alberta did not recognize the basic sciences exams of its sister province, and he had to write them again. He passed them successfully and went on in early June to take the Licentiate of the Medical Council of Canada (LMCC) exam that all doctors must pass before they can treat patients.

With the LMCC tucked in his pocket, he felt bold enough to take the next step, a pleasant one. He invited his fiancée, Editha, to join him. They had met in March 1951, during his last month of work in Baden-Baden; the daughter of a physician, she had come to the city hospital for her internship in internal medicine. Didi (as she was known) arrived in Edmonton in late June 1952, bringing to an end Otto's "dreary

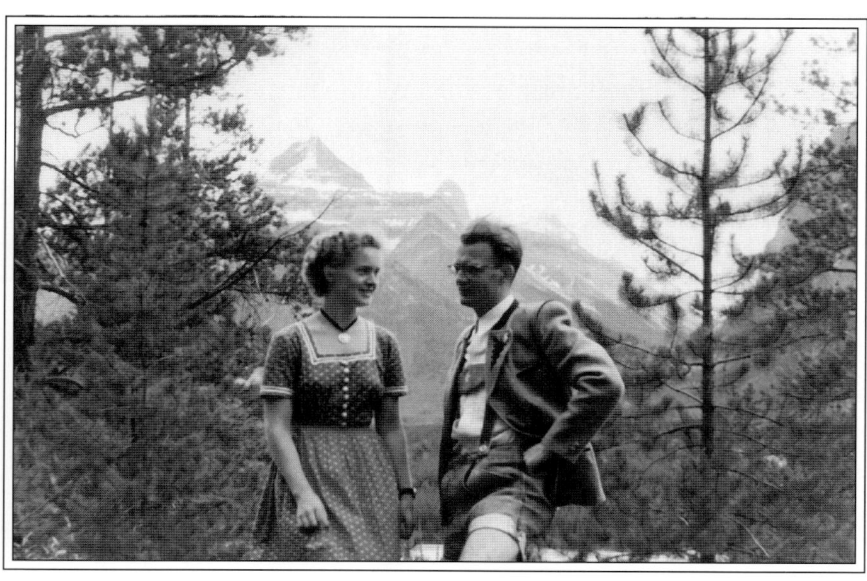

Otto and Didi in Jasper in July 1952, soon after her arrival in Canada.

life of living in the basement of the annex of the Royal Alex." They were married on July 11 and hitchhiked to Jasper Park for their honeymoon.

Didi did more than brighten Otto's life. An extraordinarily bright and talented woman, she was the ideal partner for a man who was to dedicate his life to caring for the Native people of the North. Without Didi at his side, often holding the family together, Otto could never have achieved what he did. But there was a price to pay: Didi virtually gave up her own medical career to join her adventurous fiancé in Canada. She did it willingly and gladly and was equally gracious when the time came for them to head north to face the rigours of an Arctic winter.

When it came to learning English, Didi left Otto far behind. Not only was his comprehension mediocre, but his thick accent often left listeners with a puzzled look. At a reception for the couple after Didi's arrival in Edmonton, a stranger took her aside. Nodding towards Otto, he asked: "Did that fellow just get off the boat from Germany?" She did not reply that Otto had already been in Canada for fifteen months. Otto would never succeed in shedding his German accent; but a colleague would say in years to come, "His writing is clear and precise; his use of English, in spite of his accent, is far superior to that of many for whom it is the mother tongue" (Dr. Maurice Beare, pers. comm. 1995).

During their six months together in Edmonton, Didi obtained work in the Department of Biochemistry at the University Hospital. In October 1952, Otto completed his junior internship and started work at the Charles Camsell Hospital, making it clear to his employer that he wanted to be posted to the Arctic as soon as possible. He would not have long to wait.

At that time the Camsell, with a capacity of 400 beds, received Indian and Inuit patients from many areas of the western provinces and all points of the Western Arctic. It was the ideal place to meet Native people and learn their ways—and to see firsthand some of the diseases and injuries that required them to be evacuated to Edmonton.

Otto had seen tuberculosis (TB) before, but was awestruck to see how this vicious disease had ravaged the Native population. In the early 1950s, ten percent of all Inuit were under treatment for TB in some

16 • Sunrise Over Pangnirtung

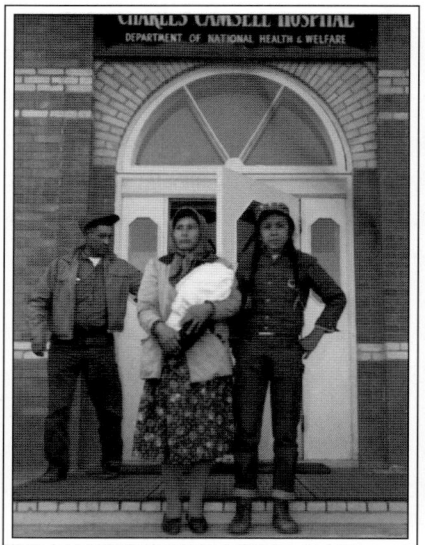 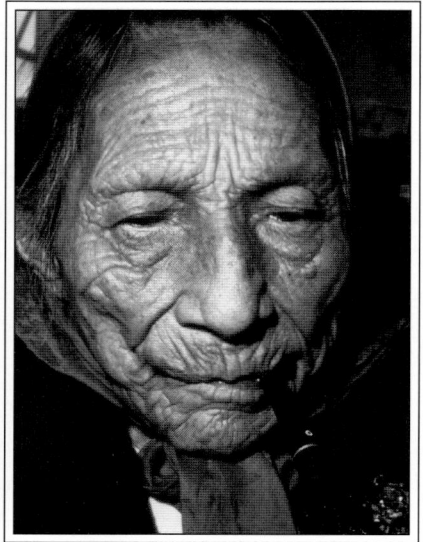

Left: Visitors from the Sunchild Cree Band near Rocky Mountain House, photographed at the main entrance to the Charles Camsell Hospital, Edmonton.

Right: Cree woman from Saskatchewan, a TB patient at the Charles Camsell Hospital in Edmonton in November 1952.

institution. Two-thirds of the Camsell's beds were filled with TB patients of all ages, pale and sickly, weak and wasted, often coughing and wheezing and bringing up blood. He saw little children with TB meningitis, one of the more dreaded forms of both diseases. He also saw cases of gunshot wounds, malnutrition, frostbite, and gangrene.

He saw children, adults, and old people, all hundreds of kilometres from their Arctic homes, and feeling out of place and lonely in the hospital, with its shiny floors, clean bedsheets, and strange food. Many were weak and racked with pain, to say nothing of homesickness. Yet they were gentle and soft-spoken, with a dignity of bearing that could not be denied. Boas (1888) had described the Inuit in similar terms, Otto remembered.

He determined to learn all he could about the health care available for the scattered residents of the Arctic and the spectrum of diseases from which they suffered. The devastation caused by TB was only too obvious, but almost as shattering were the reports of epidemics of "ordinary" childhood diseases like measles, influenza, and whooping cough that ran through the settlements like wildfire, often taking many lives.

He found out that the first nursing station in the Northwest Territories had been established by the Order of Grey Nuns in 1867, at Fort Providence near Great Slave Lake (Brett, 1969). In fact, until 1922, when the federal government posted its first physician to the Arctic, the only health care available to the Inuit had been provided by Roman Catholic and Anglican missionaries. Between 1867 and 1953, missions established health care facilities in fifteen locations. The Anglicans built the first hospital in the Northwest Territories in 1895, on the southeast coast of Baffin Island.

Dr. Leslie Livingstone, hired in 1922 as the first resident physician in the North, ended up at Pangnirtung on Baffin Island. The mission agencies had repeatedly lobbied the government for more doctors, nurses, and assistants, but it took the efforts of Dr. Frederick Banting, celebrated co-discoverer of insulin, to goad the government into action. In 1926, Banting visited his friend Livingstone at Pangnirtung and saw for himself all he needed to know. Returning to Ottawa, he commended the work of the mission hospitals but spoke in strong terms of the need for more doctors based in the North who could travel between Inuit settlements. Patients with serious illnesses would still need to be evacuated to medical facilities in the South.

Government health services in the Arctic finally shifted to high gear in 1939, when the first nursing station was opened at Fort Norman. By the time of Otto's brief period at the Camsell in 1952, about 20 nursing stations and two hospitals were in operation. All residents of the Northwest Territories were by then entitled to health care provided by the Medical Services Branch of the Department of National Health and Welfare.

The three months at the Charles Camsell Hospital gave Otto the orientation he needed to the problems of health care for the residents of Canada's North. He made the most of it. As Elva Taylor, Director of Nursing, was to say in later years: "We soon got used to the sight of the slender, young German doctor with the horn-rimmed glasses and mop of thick brown hair. He was always moving around at great speed, keen to learn all he could about the hospital, the Native patients and their health problems. Oh, he was always courteous and polite, but he never seemed to sit still. And there was an obvious earnestness of purpose about him." His English "wasn't very great," Elva reported, "but even at this early stage he seemed to build up a good rapport with the patients and to treat them with great respect." The patients, in turn, appreciated his sincere interest in them.

Otto had made it very clear to the Medical Services Branch that he wanted the earliest possible posting to the Eastern Arctic. But that was not to be, at least for a time. In January 1953, the call came to fill a desperate need in the Western Arctic: at Aklavik in the Mackenzie Delta. Otto and Didi agreed to go. The real adventure of their lives was about to begin.

4
Into the Depths of the Arctic

ON January 29, 1953 the roar of an airplane filled the skies over Aklavik, a small town on the banks of the Mackenzie River delta 175 km north of the Arctic Circle. The time was 2:00 p.m., but night was fast approaching. The temperature was -50°C.

The plane, a snub-nosed, single-engine Norseman with ski-runners, landed on the frozen river and taxied back to its bend, where a large crowd was waiting. The pilot cut the engine and opened the hatch, and out tumbled an Inuit child and a fair-haired young couple obviously from the "South." Otto and Didi Schaefer had arrived in the Arctic.

Three days before, when the venerable Norseman had lumbered into the dark sky of early morning from the runway of Edmonton's municipal airport, Otto had felt his stomach knotting up. The inside of the fuselage was already cold and cheerless, piled with boxes of freight. Instead of the usual twelve passengers, there was only one other besides themselves. She was seven-year-old Millie Chicksi, returning home after three years of treatment in the Charles Camsell Hospital for tuberculosis of the lungs and spine. She shivered so much that Otto gave her his overcoat and settled for a blanket himself.

During the flight north, the young couple from Germany kept shifting from one side of the plane to the other, entranced by the wintry landscape beneath them. The endless expanse of rolling, snow-covered hills, clumps of evergreen and bare poplar trees, frozen lakes, and flat, featureless tundra captivated them. They actually clapped their hands with joy to see the dark figures of buffalo grazing in snowy Wood Buffalo Park.

They stopped to refuel on Great Slave Lake at Yellowknife, the largest town in the Northwest Territories and a centre for gold mining since

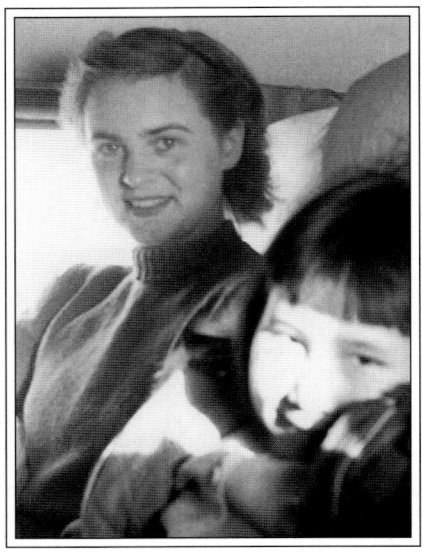

Didi Schaefer and Millie Chicksi on the plane between Edmonton and Norman Wells, on January 26, 1953. Didi served as Millie's escort on the trip.

the 1930s. Then it was on to Fort Simpson on the Mackenzie River. The river looked unimpressive in the winter, but Otto had seen pictures of the mighty Mackenzie in the summer. He estimated it to be a mile wide in some places, with large islands in the middle. He had read the biography of the famous Scottish-born explorer, Alexander Mackenzie, who in 1789 had travelled the entire 1800 km of the great river, from Great Slave Lake to the Beaufort Sea. The Mackenzie, along with the Peace and Slave Rivers, which flow into Great Slave Lake from the south, make up the longest river system in Canada (4241 km) (Marsh, 1988).

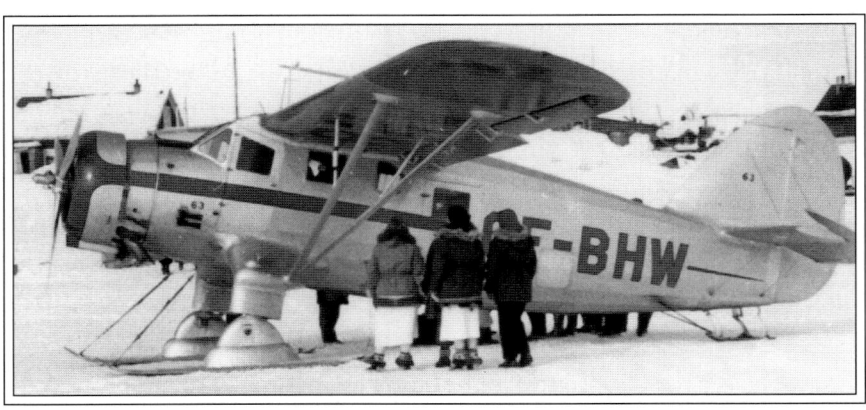

The ski-equipped aircraft in which the Schaefers made their first flight in the Western Arctic.

Coming in toward Norman Wells, a town on the east bank of the river, the passengers got their first glimpse of the Mackenzie Mountain Range to the west. They were lodged overnight in a small mobile hut that bore the grand name of "Hotel." During the unrestful night, the wind howled and roared without letup. Unfortunately, the windows and door of the hotel were not impervious to blowing snow. The Arctic blizzard raged for two full days, drifting great mounds of snow over the runway.

Finally the storm abated, and snowploughs got to work. The old Norseman coughed and sputtered, as if objecting to the sudden onset of frigid weather, but finally roared into life and took off for Aklavik. The windows soon frosted up. Otto had to scrape away the ice to get the odd glimpse of the land above the Arctic Circle. As they headed north past Arctic Red River, the great river suddenly seemed to expand into a labyrinth of loops and channels and lakes. This was the awesome Mackenzie Delta, 180 km long and 50–80 km wide. Many of the myriad islands were covered with bush and stubby little spruce trees, struggling to survive in the harshest of climates.

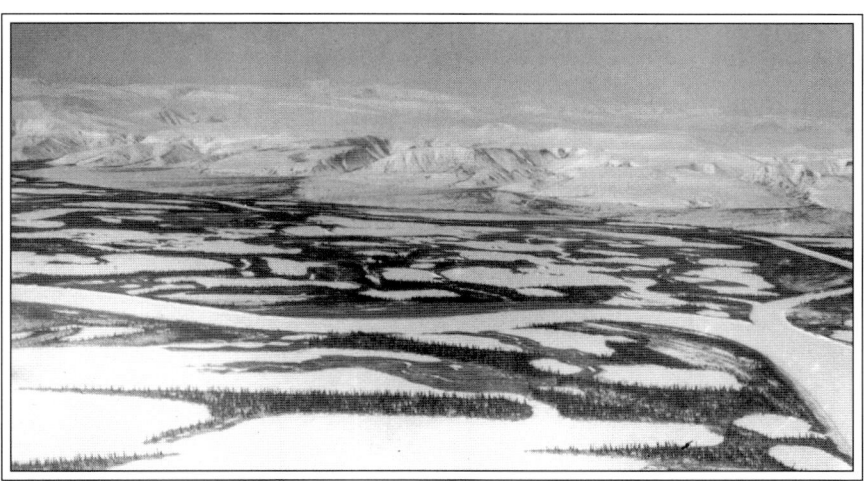

The southern part of the Mackenzie Delta, with the Richardson Mountains in the background.

Following the westernmost channel of the delta, the pilot dipped the nose of the Norseman. Turning his head and shouting above the din to his passengers, he pointed down. There, hugging a sharp curve in the river, lay the small town of Aklavik. The long, cold journey was over.

The Schaefers felt like celebrities, emerging from the little plane and being greeted by so many people. Despite the intense cold, it seemed that the whole community had come out to give them the traditional welcome. Everyone was muffled up in winter parkas with fur-trimmed hoods. Warm sealskin mitts and knee-high sealskin boots kept out the cold. Most of the women wore long "Mother Hubbard" parkas, often colourfully embroidered, that reached well below the knees. Almost immediately Otto noticed a tall, stately "Scandinavian-looking" man strolling slowly towards him in bulky caribou-skin clothing. He correctly assumed that this was Dr. Axel Laurent-Christensen, the veteran doctor he was coming to replace.

But before greeting this man, he heard an old Inuk shout, "*shik-shik!*" That started the whole crowd snickering and laughing. Otto got the distinct feeling that he was the butt of some joke. Soon everyone was singing in chorus: "*shik-shik, shik-shik!*" Later he learned that *shik-shik* ("*sik-sik*" in the Eastern Arctic) is the Inuit word for the arctic ground squirrel. Watching the newcomer emerge from the plane, taking the quick, short steps so characteristic of the man, the residents of Aklavik had quickly found an appropriate name for him. Otto never lost his distinctive gait, but a few years later the people of Cumberland Sound would give him another name: *Luttakulu* (dear little doctor).

5
Early Days at Aklavik

SEATED in the warm comfort of Dr. Axel Christensen's house after a satisfying meal of reindeer and seal meat, Otto and Didi leaned back and relaxed, the anxiety of the ordeal in the old Norseman now behind them. The 64-year-old Danish doctor had retired from the Greenland Health Service after 25 years. Then he had come to Canada's Arctic to work with what he called "real Eskimos." He seemed to enjoy Aklavik, and had worked there steadily for five years without a holiday. Otto wondered if he was getting "bushed."

Christensen's reputation as a "crusty old Dane" had reached the outside. In fact, his crustiness had culminated in a furor that led to Otto's invitation to Aklavik. A young Canadian doctor working with Christensen had criticized his senior colleague's technique during an operation. At first the operating room sizzled with venomous words, but soon the two antagonists were flinging instruments at each other. The young doctor left soon thereafter. Otto had heard both the good and the not-so-good about Dr. Christensen before leaving the Charles Camsell Hospital. He did find the old doctor somewhat difficult, but gained a respect for him. In reply to a written question from Medical Services Branch, he wrote: "He is a good man; you just have to be on the lookout for squalls."

Aklavik ("place of the grizzly bear") was the main administrative, trading, and health centre for the Western Arctic. The town had received a boost in 1920, when the Canadian Armed Forces base was moved there from Herschel Island, near the Alaskan border. Many outsiders had heard of Aklavik as the burial place of Albert Johnson, "the Mad Trapper of Rat River," who made international headlines during the winter of 1931 by killing two RCMP constables in cold blood. A posse,

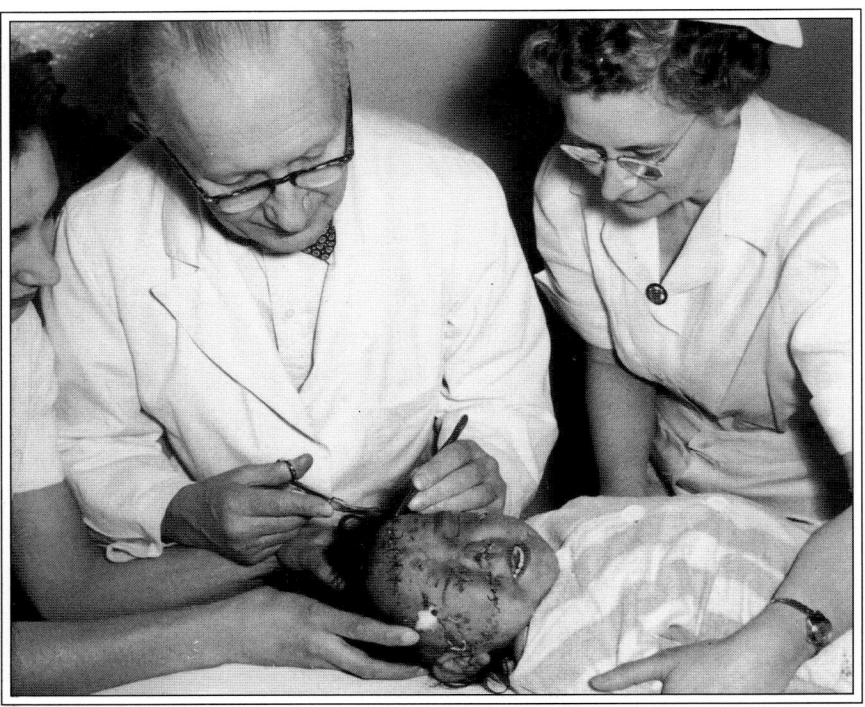

Dr. Axel L. Christensen removing sutures from the face and scalp of four-year-old Lena Pungnana, who had been badly mauled by a dog.

led by Loucheux guide Lazarus Sittichiulis, scoured the northern Yukon wilderness for over a month until they trapped the desperate fugitive. Refusing to surrender, he died in a fusillade of bullets (RCMP, 1933: 106–110). Quiet, soft-spoken Sittichiulis was still living in Aklavik when Otto arrived.

By 1953, Aklavik had 150 whites and 500 Inuit and Loucheux Indians as permanent residents, but its population doubled at muskrat hunting time in early March. Each year almost a quarter of a million muskrat pelts were taken from that vicinity. Aklavik had two hospitals, the All Saints with 110 beds and the Immaculate Conception with 50 beds. Both were busy places. At that time tuberculosis patients occupied 75 percent of the beds, leaving only 40 beds free for other patients.

Early Days at Aklavik • 25

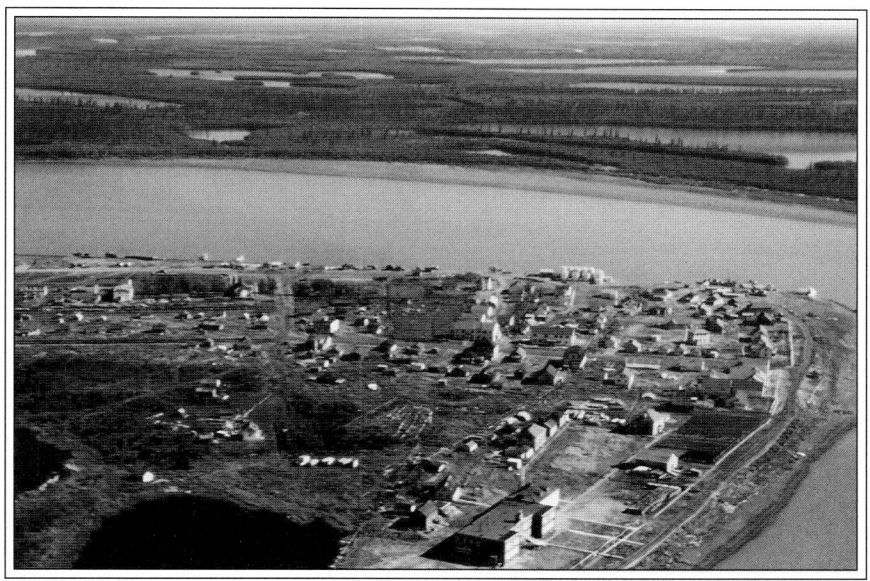

Aerial view of Aklavik in August 1954.

The workload was formidable. Besides looking after the health needs of residents, the doctors were called upon to care for 200 people in the Army Signals detachment some 3 km north of town. They also did their best to care for people living in a 500 km radius, which included Banks Island in the north and Old Crow in the Yukon. Except during times of breakup and freeze-up (each lasting two months), they travelled to hold clinics in outlying places by scheduled flights. Thick ice limited boat traffic on the Mackenzie to only four months of the year.

The two doctors worked together for three months, until Dr. Christensen left on holiday. Before his departure, a serious disagreement developed over the handling of a case. Otto invited the senior doctor to his house to discuss their differences over a cup of coffee. They did reach some accord, but Didi said later that Dr. Christensen "was a bit tempestuous and had no right to shout like that." Nonetheless, Otto was grateful to be associated with a colleague of great experience in handling the injuries and disease problems of the Inuit and Indians.

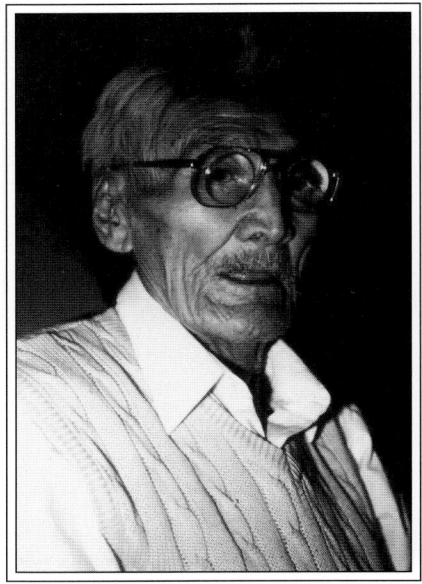 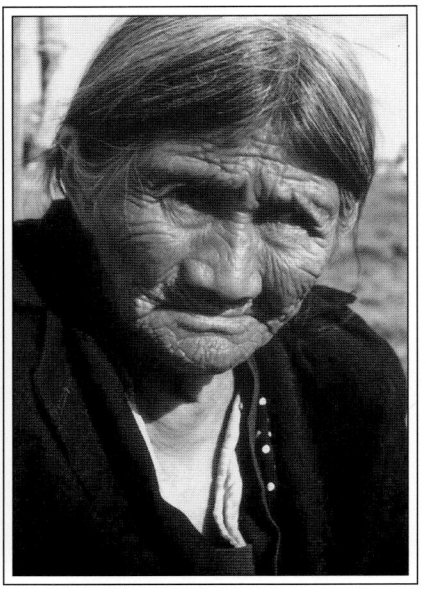

Lazarus Sittichiulis in 1989, at the age of 97. Photo by Gerald Hankins.

A Hare Indian woman who came to Aklavik in the summer of 1954 from an area north of Fort Good Hope.

After April, Otto was on his own and getting to know the people in the interesting community. The three ethnic groups, the Inuit, the Loucheux Indians, and the Hare Indians, spoke different languages, and sometimes it was difficult to tell them apart. Fortunately Otto, still striving to get his English in shape, could do his work without having to learn any of their languages: at Aklavik, even the middle-aged people spoke English. He did have trouble communicating with older people who spoke only their native tongue; luckily, most of them brought along their grandchildren when they came to the hospital.

Otto tried to learn all he could about the Inuit, who were beginning to figure prominently in his life. He observed that they were generally short in stature, thick through the torso, and had jet-black hair. The hunters among them bore the wrinkles, tanning and roughness of faces

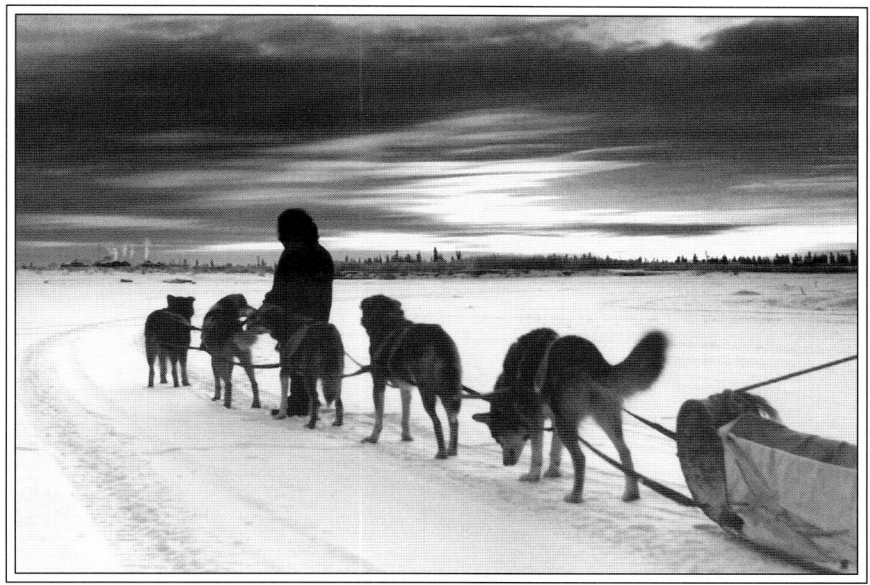

A Loucheux Indian returning from the Hudson's Bay Company store in Aklavik to his home across the Mackenzie River.

exposed to sun and icy wind blasts. Most young women wore their hair in two braids and parted down the middle. The wrinkled, weathered, character-filled faces of old people captivated Otto and made him run for his camera. Sometimes they spoke not much louder than a whisper, as though not to offend, but at other times they would laugh loudly and heartily. In time Otto would learn of their wisdom, incredible resourcefulness, and power to endure.

It amazed Otto to see how little children would accept the pain of a needle plunged into their arms for inoculation. They might whimper, but nothing more. He examined one two-year-old who had playfully licked an axe lying outside his family's tent. His mother had had to pour on hot water to separate his tongue and lips from the freezing-cold axe. The next day Otto cleaned off some of the damaged skin, a painful ordeal for the child. A tear trickled down his pudgy cheek, but he made no sound. One young man, a hunter named Napoleon, suffered with a painful hip joint, severely damaged from TB. Pus drained from his hip through two small openings in the overlying skin. In spite of the pain and the limp, he went on hunting and trapping for years. His eyes sparkled as he related to Otto the story of one "successful" hunt. He probably could have taught the more notorious Napoleon much about courage.

Meanwhile days were getting longer and warmer. By May there was hardly any darkness at all, and hours for sleeping seemed to get shorter and shorter. After months of darkness, the bright daylight hours seemed precious. Otto and Didi heard children on the swings, playing happily but noisily in the schoolyard at 2:00 a.m. They tried to cover their windows to shut out the light and get their biological rhythms in tune with the season, but it was hard to go to bed before midnight.

Spring breakup of the thick ice on the Mackenzie was one of the high points of the year. People would bet on not only the date but the

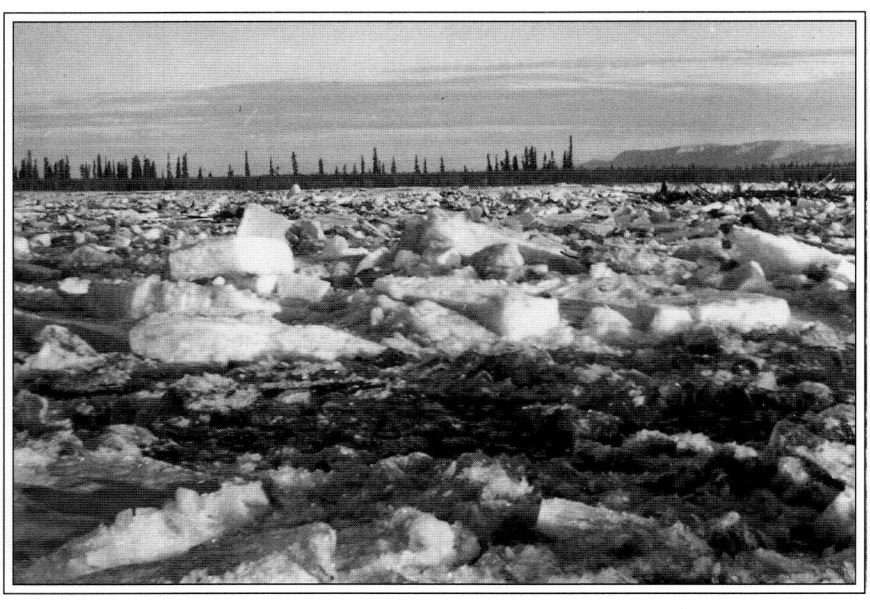

Spring breakup in the Peel Channel of the Mackenzie River on May 30, 1953.

actual time when the ice would start to move. Many stood by on the shore awaiting this dramatic moment. Long before actual breakup, the river ice was covered with several inches of meltwater. Before the massively thick ice started to move, it would rise and break up into huge chunks. It seemed to Otto that the loud crunching, grinding, and groaning was the voice of the great, imprisoned river throwing off its bondage to ice to once again gain its freedom.

One day after breakup, Otto found himself faced with a surgical problem that taxed him to the full and made him wish that the "crusty old Dane" were still around. A young American prospector had accidentally shot himself in the knee while tramping through the bush hunting. He claimed that a twig had snagged the trigger of his loaded rifle. Otto's experience at the Royal Alex had not covered this sort of challenge. But there was no way at breakup time to evacuate the patient for surgery, so he would have to do the job himself. Using spinal anaesthesia, he explored the swollen and extremely bruised knee, removed the bullet and chips of bone, and did his best to repair damaged structures. Happily, the patient made a good recovery and after a few days could walk with crutches. Otto breathed a sigh of relief. In due course the grateful patient had full mobility of his knee joint and could walk normally. Back in Seattle, he consulted with his orthopaedic surgeon, who wrote a letter to Otto commending him for the excellent surgical care given by "a specialist in internal medicine." Otto treasured that letter.

Not long afterward, he treated a young Indian who had been mauled horribly by a grizzly bear some 250 km upstream on the Peel River. Before transporting him, his companions had plastered spruce gum over the large wounds on both arms and legs and covered them with pressure dressings from their own torn shirts. When he arrived at the hospital, the man was pale and haggard but appeared to be in stable condition. An immediate transfusion replaced some of the blood he had lost. Later, in the operating room, Otto and the nurses took off the dressings on one side of his body. Then they removed all the spruce gum from those wounds, cleaned them using standard hospital antiseptics, and applied sterile dressings. It was a laborious, painstaking, and time-consuming job. When another urgent call demanded Otto's attention, he decided not to touch the remaining wounds that had been dressed by the Indians. When they changed all the dressings a week later, the wounds the Indians had treated with spruce gum were the cleanest and healing the best. In his notebook that evening, Otto made his first entry under the heading "Some Effective Traditional Folk Medicine of the North" (Schaefer, 1991). In the next few years, he would fill many pages.

6
Witness for the Prosecution

In the evening of May 10, 1953 the phone rang in the Anglican mission hospital at Aklavik. The caller asked to speak to Dr. Otto Schaefer right away. Otto was still doing his daily ward rounds. He reluctantly left the bedside of a young Inuk with tuberculosis, stuffed his stethoscope into the pocket of his white coat, and headed for the nursing station to pick up the phone. Yet another interruption in his overflowing schedule, he thought. With Dr. Christensen away, the entire workload of the Medical Officer for the Western Arctic sat heavily on Otto's willing, but relatively inexperienced, shoulders. On some days it was almost impossible to do justice to the work: caring for patients in both the Anglican and Catholic hospitals, conducting out-patient clinics, and running after emergencies. The long hours of daylight helped a little.

That phone call from RCMP Sergeant McLaughlin, police officer for the Aklavik district, would do more than interrupt his routine and complicate his busy life. In due course, it would propel him into a prominence that he would gladly have avoided. Sergeant McLaughlin had just received a call from Constable P.E. Komaiki of the detachment at Arctic Red River, a village of Loucheux Indians located on the Mackenzie River about 115 km upstream from Aklavik. Komaiki reported that the wife of Special Constable Fred Cardinal had died two days earlier from a heart attack. Cardinal, a Métis, had been working for several years as guide and interpreter for the RCMP. When Constable Komaiki had called at his home the morning after her death, Cardinal said that his 47-year-old wife had been taking pills for a heart condition.

"What would you like me to do, Sergeant McLaughlin?" asked Otto.

"Would you mind looking up the file for Mary Rose Cardinal in patient records, probably at the Catholic hospital? Then call me back as soon as you can." he replied.

Otto hastily completed his rounds, walked briskly across the village to the little Roman Catholic hospital, and searched through the files. There were several Cardinals—in fact, there were two Mary Cardinals—but fortunately only one Mary Rose Cardinal. Paging through her file, he saw one entry in his own handwriting: he had treated her for bronchitis several months before. He double-checked, but found nothing about a heart condition. *That's odd*, he thought.

When he reported his findings by phone to Sergeant McLaughlin, there was a long pause before the Mountie spoke.

"Hmm. I need to fly down to Arctic Red River tomorrow morning. I'll tell Constable Komaiki to order Cardinal not to bury his wife until I get there. Can you come with me?"

Otto frowned. "I'm extremely busy," he said. "Are you sure it's important for me to go?"

"It could be very important," said McLaughlin.

Otto agreed to go, but would not be free to leave until late in the day. Early the next evening, they landed on the small airstrip at Arctic Red River, where the first person in the crowd to greet them was Special Constable Fred Cardinal. Otto attributed his agitated state to the shock of losing his wife so suddenly. He seemed cooperative and led the Mountie and the doctor to the little Catholic church where her body had been taken. In the dim light, Otto inspected the partly frozen body, which lay in an open casket built by Cardinal from rough lumber. The two men from Aklavik conferred. Then Otto turned to Fred Cardinal.

"We need to perform an autopsy to confirm the cause of death," he said.

Cardinal scowled. "Our families and our villagers would never agree to that," he said. "Besides, we all know she had this heart problem."

"I understand," said the Mountie, "but it has to be done. Dr. Schaefer has brought his instruments and can start right now."

The church was freezing cold and too dark to do the job properly. Oblate Father Gilbert Levesque, priest at Arctic Red River, graciously offered the use of his living room. They lugged the casket over to his little house. There the doctor and the bereaved husband lifted the body of Mary Rose Cardinal out of the narrow, homemade casket onto the floor. As they did so, Otto noticed a few drops of dark blood trickling from her right ear. He held his breath for a moment, but said nothing.

When the others had absented themselves, he started the post-mortem examination. With no assistance, he painstakingly worked his way through the difficult and laborious task. Conditions were not ideal: the only light came from a flickering oil lamp and his own flashlight with weak batteries. But after completing the job more or less to his own satisfaction, Otto realized that one more task remained. Using his otoscope (an instrument for examining the ear), he peered inside the ear that had dripped blood. His heart skipped a beat. Inside the ear canal he saw tell-tale black marks that could have come only from the powder burns of a gun.

He called in Sergeant McLaughlin and whispered gravely to the RCMP officer, "I've found enough to make me suspect foul play." Then he paused, as if considering the seriousness of his words. "I need to open her skull to be absolutely sure," he continued. "I can't do that here, so we'll have to take the body on the plane back to Aklavik with us. But I

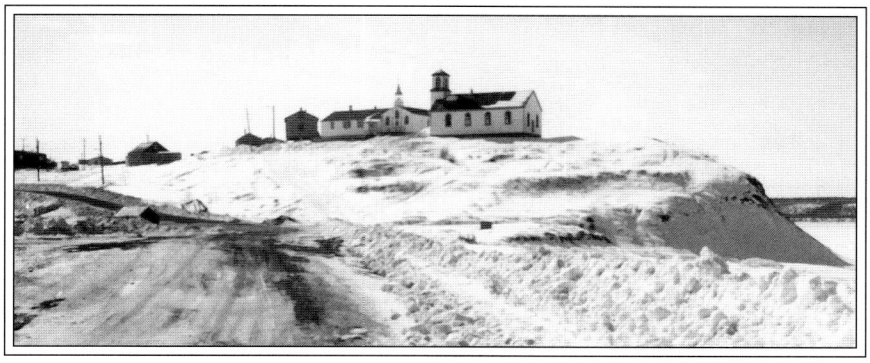

The chapel (with spire) and Catholic Church at Arctic Red River, May 1987. Photo by Gerald Hankins.

think we have enough evidence for you to arrest Fred Cardinal." The RCMP man arrested Cardinal on the spot and took him into custody.

Back at Aklavik the following day, working under better conditions, Otto Schaefer completed the unpleasant but important part of the autopsy. He opened the skull of the unfortunate woman. It came as no surprise to find a path of destruction and bone slivers leading from the ear across the lower part of the brain to the opposite side of the skull. From that point, he extracted with his forceps a .22 bullet.

Fred Cardinal was tried twice for the first-degree murder of his wife. The first trial, held in a school room in Aklavik, started on July 9, 1953 and lasted three days. Even old-timers in the Northern Mackenzie district had never heard of anything quite so sensational happening in their area. For the entire three days, the school premises swarmed with people. Children were not allowed to enter the actual room during the proceedings, but they jammed together outside, noses flattened against the windows and eyes wide with excitement.

As a key witness for the prosecution, Otto was called upon to testify and to present the report of his post-mortem examination of the body of Mary Rose Cardinal. His findings were indisputable. But had he not taken the trouble to open the skull of the deceased woman to find the bullet, Cardinal and his lawyer might have got away with their own version of the story—that Cardinal had poked a stick in his wife's ear to ease the pain of an earache.

Fred Cardinal was found guilty and sentenced to hang on October 10, 1953. But when the defence learned that a psychiatrist enlisted to examine the accused was not a properly qualified psychiatrist and therefore not an "expert witness," a mistrial had to be declared. A second trial was scheduled for January 1954 in Yellowknife.

On January 8, court was held in the Caribou Room of the Ingraham Hotel, Yellowknife, with Mr. Justice Boyd McBride presiding (*News of the North*, January 8, 1954:1). This time, Cardinal admitted under questioning that he had shot his wife in the ear while she lay sleeping. Once again a jury found him guilty, and he was sentenced to death. He was hanged at Fort Smith, then capital of the Northwest Territories, in April 1954—one of the last persons to be hanged in Canada.

The drama was over, but questions remained. With Cardinal on the scaffold, was justice honoured and wrong redressed? Otto Schaefer could have felt legitimate satisfaction with his major role in a court case that saw a murderer paying the price for his crime. But he regretted that another life had to be taken to settle the matter. It bothered him—and others—to learn that another player in the tragedy had got off scot-free. Some weeks later, while visiting Arctic Red River, he heard the astounding news from several Loucheux Indians that "a certain seductive woman in the village," as they described her, had persuaded Fred to kill his wife. But she was no longer around. Fearing that her life was in danger from friends in sympathy with Fred Cardinal, village authorities had whisked her off the scene. She was last known to be in the protective care of Catholic nuns at Fort Resolution on Great Slave Lake.

7
Patients and Characters

THE long daylight hours of summer produced an explosion of growth in the fertile Mackenzie Delta. Flowers of deep burgundy red and vivid aquamarine blue blossomed in profusion, waving in the warm breeze. Pink and mauve moss campion hugged the rocks. But what impressed Otto and Didi most were the vegetables that seemed to grow before their eyes. In the garden of Father Binamé, director of the Immaculate Conception Hospital, they saw cabbages bigger than soccer balls.

On August 11, 1954, the temperature at Tuktoyaktuk on the Beaufort Sea was 27.2°C, warm enough to entice Otto and others to go swimming. After a few brisk moments immersed in the chilly water of the harbour at Tuk (as they called it), they could claim to have been swimming in the Arctic Ocean.

Otto was one of the passengers who had travelled downstream from Aklavik on the Anglican mission boat, the *Messenger*. He remembers the birds that flew out from the bushes as the boat putt-putted its way northward through the labyrinth of lakes and channels. Abundant ducks and geese grazed on the fresh weeds and grass along the edges. He saw two ospreys winging overhead and a falcon perched on a fallen tree. Swallows flitted through the clouds of mosquitoes that hung over the water. Fortunately, the boat was moving forward fast enough to elude the blood-hungry Arctic marauders.

At Tuk Otto examined Charlie Gruben, a boy who, after striking his head on the ice several weeks before, had developed weakness of the right side of his body. He walked like an old man paralyzed by a stroke. Otto wondered if the head injury might have left a clot of blood inside his skull. The clot could be pressing on that part of the brain that activated the movement of his right arm and leg.

To solve the problem meant seeking the skill of a specialist, so Otto arranged for Charlie to catch the next flight to Edmonton. At the Charles Camsell hospital, a neurosurgeon found and removed the offending clot of blood. The boy came back to Tuk and was soon walking normally again.

Apart from his clinical condition, Otto was intrigued with the boy's racial background: both his parents were offspring of American whalers and Inuit women. Around the turn of the century, whaling had been one of the largest industries in North America. Whalers from Scotland and the United States (in particular the eastern seaboard) took great numbers of whales from Alaska and the Mackenzie Delta, as well as from southern Baffin Island in the Eastern Arctic. The whalers relied heavily on the Inuit for help and all too often exploited them. As Otto worded it, whalers also "widened the genetic base" of the local inhabitants, sometimes with the benefit of marriage, but often not.

In the course of their exploits, the whalers frequently left a sordid trail of misery and woe. In the early 1900s, Kittigazuit, 32 km west of Tuk, was a thriving settlement of Delta Inuit. A few years later it was completely deserted. Dr. R.S. MacNeish, archaeologist from the National Museum in Ottawa, visited the site and examined human bones. He and others came to the conclusion that viral epidemics (from contact with outsiders) and decimation of the whale population had caused the death of 90 percent of its 1000 residents.

Norma Westgate, a graduate nurse from Toronto General Hospital, was already on duty at the Anglican Hospital when Otto and Didi arrived in Aklavik. She had heard the *shik-shik* story and found that it was indeed hard to keep up with the trim, fast-stepping doctor on ward rounds. She remembers his dedication to the patients and "his always stopping to scribble something in a little notebook." "He wanted to know the whys and wherefores of everything and was prepared to learn from everyone," she said.

The questioning, searching, note-taking, and pondering would be the pattern for the rest of his life. It was not enough to care for sick patients—he wanted to learn about their families, their homes, the

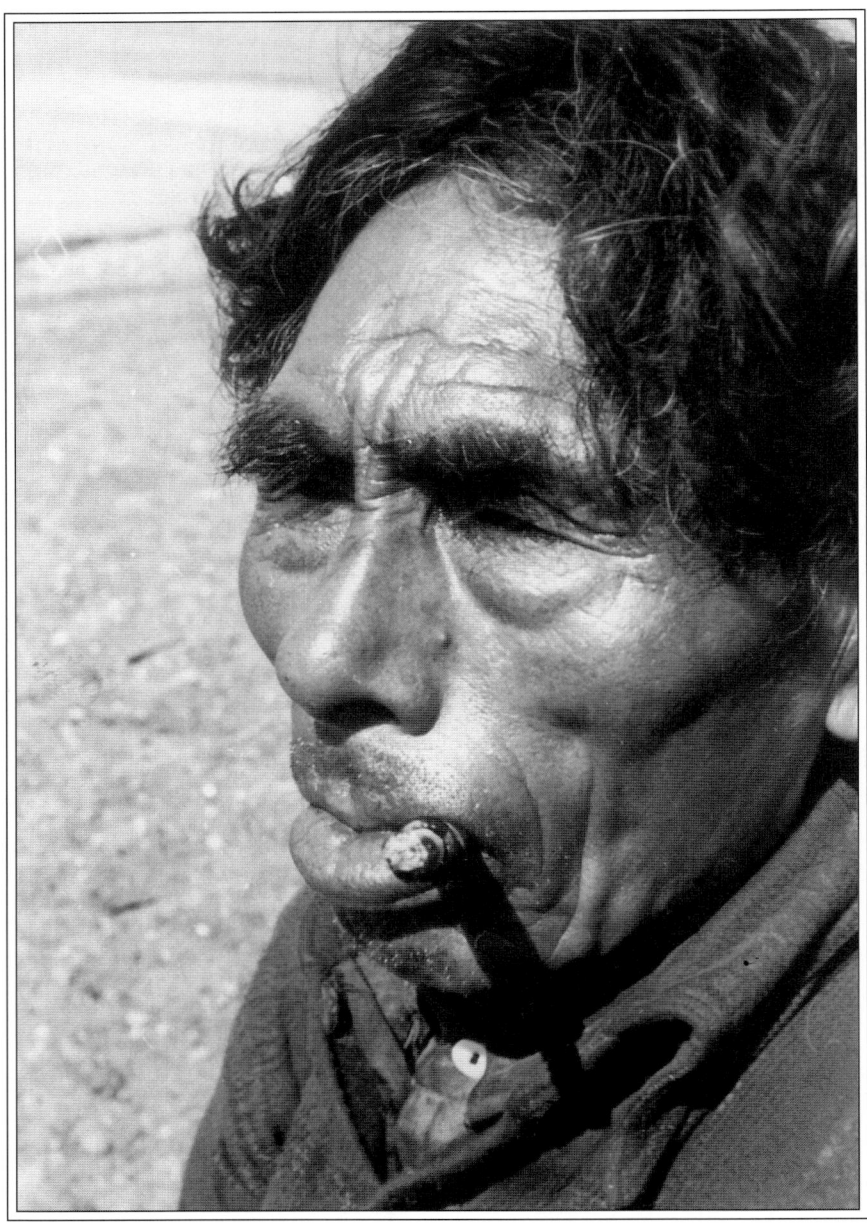

Maurice Pokiak, a survivor from Kittigazuit, met by Otto Schaefer in Tuktoyaktuk in 1953.

possible causes of their illnesses, and whether others in the community suffered from them. He would soon broaden his interests to include such subjects as epidemiology, a science that studies the spread and the incidence of disease. As Norma said, "He sincerely felt that much more needed to be done for the health of the Inuit, without ruining their way of life."

An opportunity soon arose to conduct a little study. Otto had noticed that the Native children attending the residential school often had to leave class with nosebleeds. Some bleeds started from vigorous nose-blowing, but others occurred spontaneously. It puzzled him. He decided then to do a survey of children living at home in huts and tents, where the air was never as warm as in the schools, but usually more humid. They rarely got nosebleeds. He concluded that the school's central heating of the cold Arctic air produced such dryness of the nasal passages that the delicate tissue cracked and bled. Simple humidification of the heated air solved the problem.

After Dr. Christensen returned from holiday, Otto felt more free to visit some of the scattered settlements within reach by plane or boat. He will never forget one 24-hour foray to the village of Old Crow, a remote isolated village on the Porcupine River in northwest Yukon. No doctor had seen the residents, mostly Loucheux Indians, for two years. Veteran pilot Mike Zubko landed his small plane on the makeshift sandbar landing strip after an early morning flight. No sooner had the spinning propeller come to rest than the plane was surrounded with people. This time Otto had brought along two willing helpers, Didi and Norma Westgate. He trundled out the portable x-ray machine, set it up, and got to work in the local schoolhouse.

All 140 residents of Old Crow got the benefit of some medical help. Didi inoculated the children and Norma took x-rays, while Otto did physical examinations, gave out medicines, pulled teeth, and fitted people with glasses. They worked all day. But it wasn't supposed to be all work. The villagers, determined to be hospitable, had made plans for a dance that was, of course, to include the guests.

At 2:00 a.m., a young man, fiddle in hand, appeared at the schoolhouse: "Aren't you coming to the dance?" he asked. "We're all

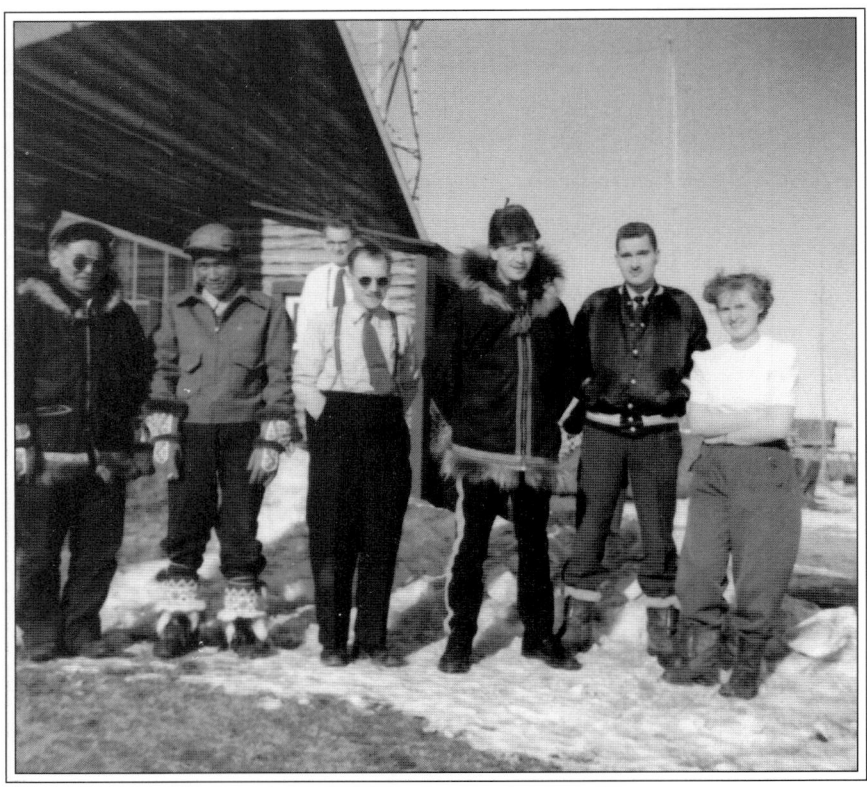

Otto and Didi Schaefer visiting Old Crow on April 23, 1954. From left to right stand two residents of Old Crow, the schoolteacher (an Anglican missionary), two RCMP officers, and Didi. Otto is standing behind the schoolteacher. Photo by Norma Westgate.

waiting for you." The two ladies nodded. Off they went, to dance as they never had before. Otto kept plugging away until 5:00 a.m. before joining the crowd. Somehow his flagging energy revived on the dance floor. They danced until 7:00, when sleepless Mike Zubko appeared: "We've got to head back," he said. And they made it back to Aklavik, just 24 hours after leaving, in time to start another day's work.

Like many frontier towns, Aklavik had, besides its "ordinary" people, a group of "irregulars." Most of the latter were outright eccentric or had a strange story to tell. Otto was called once to the home of Mike Jacobsen, a slight elderly man, and Vera, his rather substantial Inuit wife. Jacobsen, born in Latvia, was part-German and part-Swedish. He had run away from home at the age of 14 and eventually joined a whaling fleet operating out of Massachusetts. After the sharp decline of whaling around 1910, he had started trapping white foxes near Baillie Island, about 200 km northeast of Tuktoyaktuk.

One day, Mike accidentally shot himself in the left hand. Infection from the ugly wound spread into his arm. He lay in his

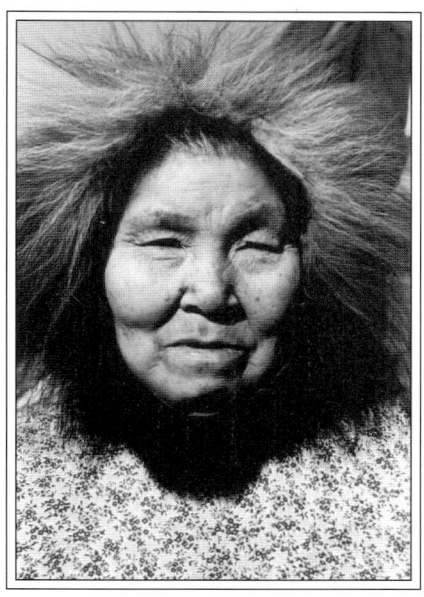

Mrs. Vera Jacobsen.

little hut, weak, feverish, parched with thirst, and ready to die. A 16-year-old Inuit girl from a local family group somehow heard of his plight and came to his hut. With a knife, she cut open the huge red abscess in his arm and sucked out the pus. She nursed him back to health and undoubtedly saved his life. As Jacobsen told it later, "She certainly did save my life, and the least I could do was to marry her!" It had turned out, Otto noticed, to be a fruitful marriage in more ways than one.

Of all the strange and colourful characters calling Aklavik their home, old Joe Veitch stood alone, in Otto's opinion. During the summer of 1953, he confronted the 84-year-old giant of a man for the second time at the door of his one-room shack by the river. Previously old Joe, seeing Otto struggling to lug his canoe through deep mud down to the river one evening, had come to his aid. "First he carried the canoe, then me, down to the river," said Otto.

Joe claimed to have served in the Boer War and to have come to Aklavik 50 years before. His brown, weather-beaten face, tousled head,

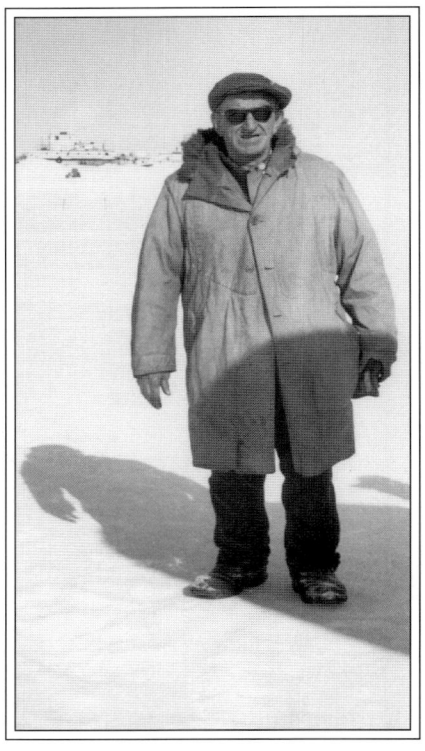

Joe Veitch in Aklavik, April 1953.

and fog-horn voice reminded Otto of a great bull moose. Joe Veitch was a law unto himself, as Otto quickly found out. For one thing, he had gained a reputation for borrowing things from his friends "on a long-term basis." During World War II, Joe had worked on the Alaska Highway and on the side, made home brew and distilled whisky. Caught once by the RCMP, he was kept locked up in custody until he could pay a hefty fine. To the surprise of the police, he did pay the fine after a couple of weeks, thanks to the helping hand of his American "customers."

Otto sent Joe to Edmonton for cataract surgery and was quite surprised when he returned a week later, still with his cataracts. Otto asked what had gone wrong. It turned out that several young doctors in white coats had come along and looked into Joe's eyes with bright lights. It was more than he could stand. "They weren't going to make a guinea pig out of me," he humphed. He walked out of the hospital, made his way to the airport, and after two days boarded a plane for the North, without a ticket. No one dared stand in his way.

Joe was well known for the dog team he kept outside and for several cats that shared his dirty little shack with him. At the time of Otto's visit, a cat and four kittens were ensconced on the grey sheets of his unmade bed. On the kitchen table, two other cats were licking up leftovers. Otto mentioned casually what the cats were doing and got a gruff reply. "What's wrong with that?" he growled. "If it wasn't for my cats, I'd have to wash the dishes." After examining Joe, Otto was on the point of leaving when the patient offered him some of his home brew. "Thanks very much," said Otto. "Maybe next time."

8
Didi and the Arctic

FREED from having to learn a new language in Aklavik, Otto and Didi were determined to get to know the people. It was inconceivable that they not mingle with their Indian and Inuit neighbours, not meet with them socially at community affairs, not invite them home to dinner. True, some "southerners" lived apart—and sometimes aloof—but not the Schaefers. Jack Grainge, regional engineer for the entire Northwest Territories, was amazed at Otto's sweeping knowledge of the whole community. The two attended many meetings together. Jack remembers his "ready and gentle wit" and his "genuine interest in the Native people."

Otto had taken his enterprising wife not only to Old Crow but also to Tuk and Fort McPherson on the Peel River. Eventually she got to all the settlements in the Northern Mackenzie district except for Sachs Harbour on Banks Island. Whenever there was time after taking blood specimens for lab tests and inoculating children, she would make friends with the local people. Kenneth Pililuk and his wife Sarah, who lived at an old whaling station about 16 km west of Tuk, became her good friends. On the next boat trip downstream, Otto arranged for Didi to stay with them for a few days.

Didi was also a gracious hostess in her own home, always willing to accept guests even if they appeared unannounced or in the company of her husband who "had forgotten" to warn her. She could take bold ventures with her cooking too, as Jack Grainge found out one night. Invited to dinner, Jack noticed a strange but not unpleasant smell of meat cooking as he entered the Schaefer home. He made no enquiries, but before Otto began carving the odd-looking roast in front of him, Jack's curiosity got the better of him. Otto saw his puzzled look. "Never had muskrat before?" he asked. Jack admitted that he hadn't. Otto went on to explain to the newcomer that Aklavik was one of the richest

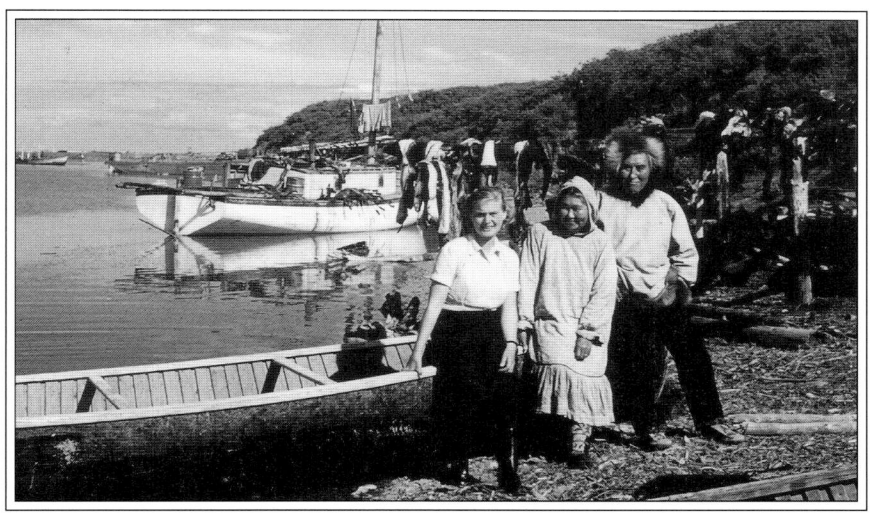

Didi with friends Kenneth and Sarah Pililuk at Whitefish Station, a beluga whaling camp west of Tuktoyaktuk.

trapping grounds for muskrat on the continent. At one time, when ladies' fur coats were fashionable, the pelts had sold for $2.50, but now they were worth only 65 cents. "But the meat hasn't decreased in value," he said. "Would you like to try some? If not, we prepared some roast beef for you, just in case." Jack not only enjoyed the hospitality that night, but he actually liked the muskrat. In later years he related that "it wasn't bad at all."

Didi was beginning to love the Arctic, enjoying each of the highly contrasting winter and summer seasons. But her warm feelings might easily have turned to loathing after a terrifying, life-threatening day in June 1953. She had agreed to escort a group of a dozen children travelling upstream to join their families at Arctic Red River (scene of the Cardinal murder episode) and Fort Good Hope. Father Binamé of cabbage fame had asked her to go along. They travelled in the cabin of a barge pulled by a motorboat. Also aboard were two nuns and an Indian, the boat's pilot. They left about 10:00 p.m., expecting to reach Arctic Red River by 6:00 the following morning.

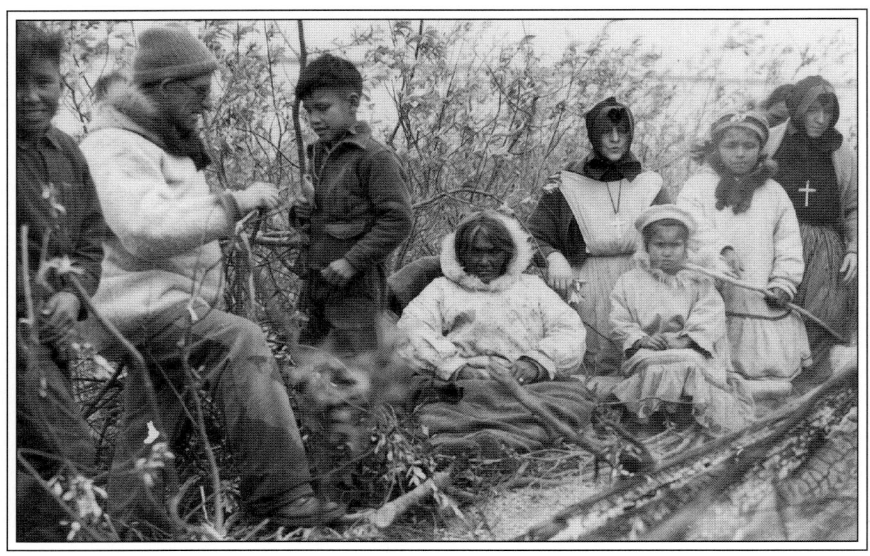

Father Binamé with schoolchildren and nurses from the Roman Catholic Hospital, in the bush after the storm. Photo by Didi Schaefer.

It was a beautiful, peaceful trip until they reached Point Separation, where the Mackenzie splits into many channels. Suddenly they were hit by a "hurricane-like storm" blowing down from the North. (Otto later reported that trees around Aklavik were torn up by the roots.) Didi had the feeling that the flat barge would break up. The gale flung the small motorboat against the barge with a terrible crash. Risking his life, Father Binamé succeeded in separating the two, and dropped the barge's anchor. But the heaving waves and brutal wind snapped the cable, and the barge drifted into the muddy shore. In the churning, choppy water of the raging river, all the children and both sisters got seasick. Water gushed into the barge's cabin, threatening to drown them all. Didi and Father Binamé bailed for all they were worth.

Finally the storm abated. They hopped off the barge into knee-deep water and mud and made their way ashore, carrying blankets and sleeping bags over their heads. Didi's diary (excerpted in Schaefer, 1953) described what happened next:

The Indian school children were a delight—on land in the bush, they were in their element. Under Father Binamé's direction, they cleared an area of bush and started a large fire to dry their clothes. The boys climbed on the stranded barge, got their reindeer meat and bread, etc., and started a meal. I sure enjoyed the meal they offered me. We felt sorry for the Indian pilot and the Oblate brother who had remained on the cabin boat for 24 hours with no food. The wind was still too strong to pull up their two anchors and come over to us...

We prepared places to sleep away from the smoke of the fire and settled down. But Fr. Binamé soon woke us up saying the storm had died down and the cabin boat was heading our way. It took another couple of hours to get the barge out of the mud bank, but by 3:00 a.m. we were on our way.

We got to Arctic Red River by 6:00 a.m. and found that the storm had caused trouble there too, tearing the balcony off the mission house. But the sight of happy parents taking their children in their arms is something I would never have missed.

9
Shamans and Missionaries

CHRISTIAN missionaries entered the far-flung regions of the North primarily to offer education and health care. It is perhaps understandable that many Inuit were drawn towards the faith of these men and women who dedicated their lives to serve them.

Inuit religion before that time was a mixture of spirits and magic (Farb, 1968). The Inuit lived in a world where the central concerns were survival and the ever-present search for food. Spirits controlled much of their lives, and they did their best to placate the spirits. They believed that illness of body or mind could be caused by an evil spirit, or by sin (usually the breaking of a taboo), or by the witchcraft of a malevolent shaman (spirit intermediary). But not all shamans did harm. They moved freely in the supernatural world and contended with the spirits on their own ground. In times of illness, the family of the sick person might call the *angakok* (shaman) and offer a gift, hoping that he could exert a favourable influence on the evil spirit.

Before he became a Christian while attending the Anglican Mission School at Hay River, Cyril Wingek, a Mackenzie Delta Inuk, had held such beliefs. He thought that the *angakok* could communicate with the spirits of dead people, animals, insects, and even the elements. Cyril told Otto a story about the Inuit belief in spirits that inhabit the natural world. One summer when Cyril was visiting the Coppermine area, black clouds gathered and thunder and lightning kept coming closer. He watched an old man fitting an arrow into his bow, ready to fire into the thunder clouds.

"When are you going to shoot?" asked Cyril.

"I'll wait until they're overhead. Then I'll get them," he said.

When a peal of thunder roared right above them, the old man pulled back on the bow as hard as he could and let fly. His arrow shot high into the air, but not quite high enough to strike the angry thunderclouds. It landed back on the ground a few yards from them. Cyril asked his friend if he had hit anything.

"I don't know," he said, "but I'm pretty sure I scared them off."

Cyril was about 60 when Otto treated him for tuberculosis in the All Saints Hospital at Aklavik. He was a superb storyteller, having learned the art when travelling as a missionary to the Central Arctic, soon after his conversion. He wanted to tell others about the new-found faith that gave him such freedom, he said. But in Bathurst Inlet, he found that few people would listen to him and the Bible stories he liked to tell. He got discouraged. One day a bright idea came: he would learn all the stories in the book of Grimm's fairy tales

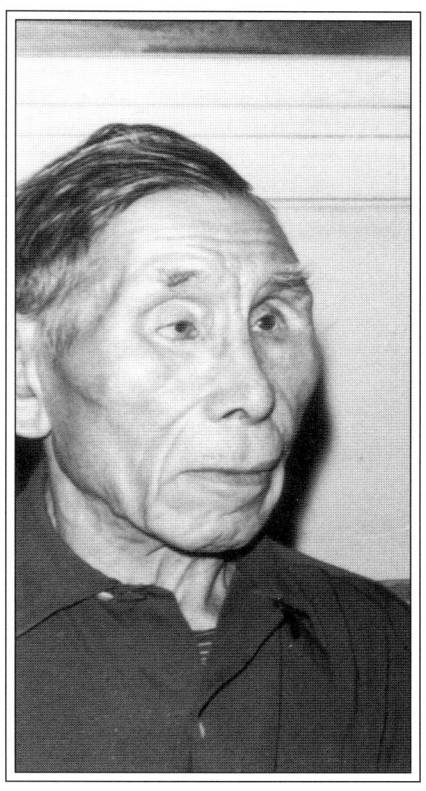

Cyril Wingek.

that he had brought from Hay River. He did just that, and found that the fairy tales captivated his listeners so completely that he could gradually switch over to Bible stories and still hold their attention.

Otto developed a great deal of respect for the directors of the two hospitals that served as his workshops in Aklavik. Father Binamé ran the 50-bed Immaculate Conception Hospital and a 100-pupil school, with the help of an assistant priest, 4 brothers, and 17 nuns. A gentle but powerful man, he could lug a 100-pound pack on his back. Archdeacon J. Harold Webster was no less remarkable. Like Father Binamé, he ran a large hospital and a 100-pupil school. At the All Saints "Cathedral," he conducted the English services while the Reverend

50 • Sunrise Over Pangnirtung

James Sittichinli, a Loucheux Indian, led worship in the Loucheux language.

While in the Central Arctic, Archdeacon Webster had travelled hundreds of kilometres annually to visit outlying mission stations. On

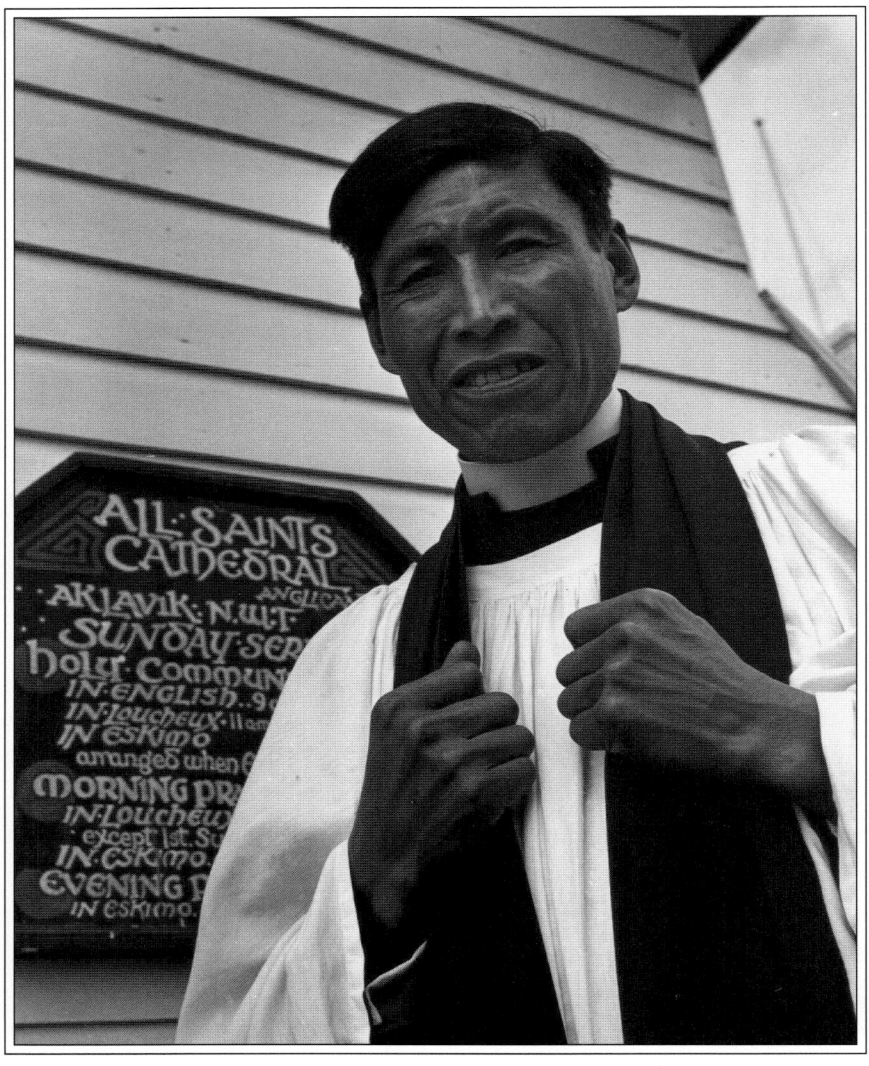

The Reverend James Sittichinli. Photo by George Hunter.

one of these trips, his dogs saved him from almost certain death. He was travelling to a seal camp only 19 km away from Coppermine when a blizzard closed in on him. Surrounded by whirling snow, he could not even see his own feet. Somehow his lead dog got unhitched. While he was struggling to retrieve him, the other dogs ran off with the sled. Webster wandered around, hopelessly lost, and finally dug a deep hole in the snow and waited for rescue—or the end. Meanwhile his dogs instinctively ran through the blizzard back to Coppermine, alerting his friends that he was missing. But it took three full days before they found him, barely clinging to life.

Binamé and Webster both shunned the idea of competition. True, on one occasion while broadcasting on the Aklavik radio station, they got into such an argument about a finer point of the faith that the local Signal Corps temporarily cut off the transmission. But such disputes were rare. Both realized they worked for the same Lord in the same "vineyard," where the demands and challenges demanded the best of them and left no time for rivalry.

10

The Final Months at Aklavik

OTTO and Didi Schaefer had together faced many of the hazards of the North—frostbite, hypothermia, isolation, and strange food—and survived unscathed. Apart from weariness and fatigue, the medical work did Otto no real harm. But for three weeks in March 1953 he suffered excruciating pain. One day, after lifting a 50-pound barrel of aviation gas into Mike Zubko's plane, he felt a nagging pain in his lower back. Lifting barrels wasn't part of his job description; he had just wanted to help. He tried to ignore the backache, but by the next day, the pain and stiffness were so bad that he had to walk like a lame duck. Later the pain shot down his leg into his right foot. He tried his best to keep going, taking pain-relieving pills to make life bearable. But with Dr. Christensen away, he needed help. The Department of Health and Welfare sent up Dr. Greenidge from Edmonton.

Otto consulted by phone with former associates at the Charles Camsell Hospital and later with a neurosurgeon from the University Hospital. The consultant diagnosed a ruptured inter-vertebral disc pressing on nerve roots and advised operation without delay. Otto hoped he was wrong. On April 5 he had to fly to Norman Wells to hold a clinic, backache or no backache. It was a rough flight through storm clouds. Turbulence shook the old Norseman so severely that Otto thought his back would break. He tried everything and finally slithered off the hard bench onto the floor, where he rolled up into the foetal position with a sleeping bag wrapped around him. Suddenly the plane gave a tremendous lurch. Miraculously, Otto got instant relief from his pain. He could hardly believe it. When they landed at Norman Wells, he could stand up straight and walk normally for the first time in three weeks. It was dramatic relief.

After cancelling the proposed surgery, Otto told Dr. Greenidge he could return to Edmonton, but asked if before leaving he would put him in a body cast of plaster of Paris. Otto wore this cast for two months, giving his back the time to "stabilize." Otto never had to endure such pain again, but he was left with what he called a "ramrod-stiff lower lumbar spine." Didi made sure that he did not lift any more barrels of aviation gas.

Before leaving Aklavik, Otto found himself involved in decisions for the future of the little town. Curt Merrill, a town planner and geologist hired to search for "alternative locations," explored the east side of the Delta by helicopter in April 1954. No one could deny the present site had problems. Every year the river flooded parts of the town, and thawing of the unstable ground caused houses to heave and shift. After breakup, the thick mud along the river bank almost blocked people from getting to their boats. But these were not the real reasons for choosing another site to replace Aklavik as trading and administrative centre for the Western Arctic. It irked Otto to hear national CBC quoting him as advocating the move:

> *Dr. Schaefer convinced General Young that no safe and hygienic drinking water and sewage disposal conditions existed in the present location of Aklavik in the muddy Delta with its unstable and shifting riverloops and lakes.* (quoted in Schaefer, 1954)

He had said no such thing, and it bothered him to be misquoted. What the U.S. Defence Department really wanted was a place with solid soil and gravel to build an airport for the Air Force and a site for the proposed DEW (Distant Early Warning) line radar stations that would warn against a possible invasion by the Soviet Union. Inuvik on the east side of the Delta would be built to serve that purpose. Construction of the massive DEW-line stations in several locations in 1955 started the chain of events that would change the life of the North forever.

With September's first snow came the realization that Otto and Didi would soon say good-bye to Aklavik. Their two-year term was coming to an end. They would take away with them a host of good memories, new skills and experiences, and lasting friendships. But they would take more—"something" that personified Aklavik for them for years to come—a son, Lothar, born on October 15, 1953. The Aklavik assignment had definitely been a second choice for them, a job to be done and a niche to be filled until they could get to Cumberland Sound on Baffin Island, which they called "the land of Franz Boas." Didi expressed their feelings after their departure:

> *We found the Western Arctic and Subarctic with their Eskimo and Indian as well as non-native trappers so interesting that we were sorry we had to leave. The last summer and fall were so beautiful for both of us that we would have loved to stay and felt homesick for the land and people there from the moment we left.* (quoted in Schaefer, 1953)

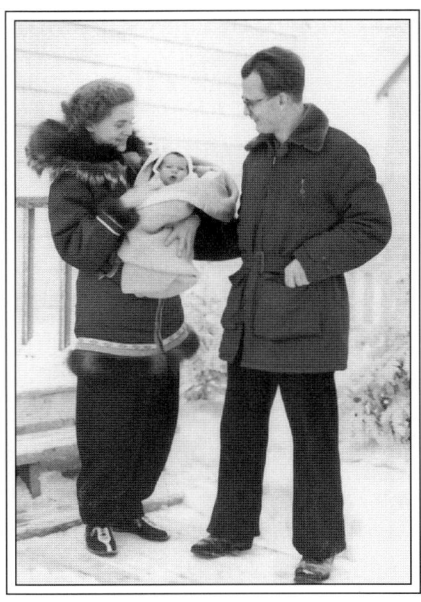

As he had done on that cold January day when they landed on the river ice, Dr. Christensen, the "crusty old Dane," invited them to his home: their final meal was a goose he had shot himself. But it wasn't over yet. On September 28, the day before their planned departure, a foot of snow fell. Otto joined the party of volunteers, shovelling to clear a runway on the frozen mud flats in front of the Anglican residential school. It was hard work. Surprisingly, his back stood up well. But when the plane

Otto and Didi with their eight-week-old son Lothar in December 1953. Photo by Annie Andreason.

flew overhead, Otto signalled to the pilot to do a few more circuits. The snow-shovellers hadn't quite finished their work.

The townspeople gathered around the plane to say good-bye to the red-faced, panting doctor and his wife and baby. Most had already stopped by their home to say thanks and farewell during the last few days. Even old Joe Veitch was there with his dogs. They climbed aboard, and soon the little plane was skimming over the snowy landing strip, leaving a slipstream of fine snow to drift down on their waving friends.

11
On Board the *C.D. Howe*

Standing on deck I saw a mighty iceberg-plateau riding high out of the water about 5 km from our ship; it must have broken off from the Greenland ice cap at Melville Bay or Humboldt glacier....

So wrote Otto Schaefer on board the *C.D. Howe*, steaming north up the Labrador coast on a frosty September evening in 1955. Almost instinctively he thought of the "unsinkable" luxury liner *Titanic*, which had struck just such a monstrous iceberg on April 14, 1912. Water had gushed in through a huge 90-metre gash, and within three hours the *Titanic* had sunk in the frigid water of the Labrador Stream, taking over 1500 human lives with her.

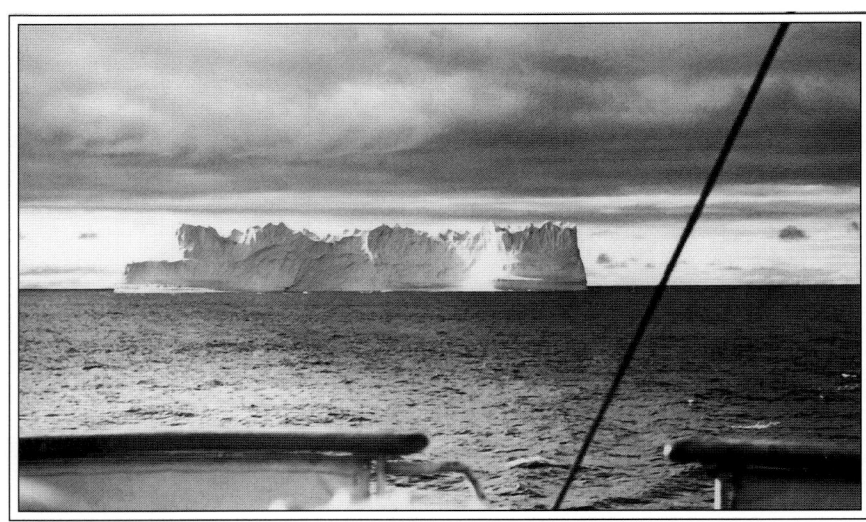

Iceberg in Davis Strait.

On June 24, Otto and Didi and their family (they now had two sons, Lothar and Alfred) had boarded the *C.D. Howe* in Montreal for its annual "Eastern Arctic Patrol." Over the next two months, their floating home would stop at a score of settlements from Hudson Bay up to Grise Fiord on Ellesmere Island in the High Arctic. A semi-icebreaker, the *C.D. Howe* carried supplies for northern residents and offered medical care. For many, it was the only medical care likely to come their way.

Otto's job as the ship's medical officer was to examine patients at every settlement. But before the *C.D. Howe* returned to home base in Montreal in September, the Schaefer family would disembark at one of its last ports of call, the hamlet of Pangnirtung on Baffin Island's Cumberland Sound. There Otto would begin a two-year term as Medical Officer for the Eastern Arctic.

Pang, as they called it, had been his first choice all along, something he had made very clear to his employer, the Medical Services Branch. He and Didi knew it to be an isolated, frontier settlement—far different from Aklavik—but they had their hearts set on going there. Otto welcomed the Eastern Arctic tour as an opportunity to examine and study the great variety of Inuit patients that would come to see the doctor at every port of call. But he longed equally to see Canada's rugged and unfriendly eastern seaboard. Like many Europeans, he had read about the 400-year-long search for the "Northwest Passage" that would allow ships to sail through the Canadian Arctic Archipelago to India and China. Names like Davis, Parry, Hudson, and Rae were not new to him. The story of Sir John Franklin's tragic expedition of 1845 still burned in his memory. He would soon have the opportunity to see the islands, bays, and channels that bore the names of these past heroes, and to relive their adventures in the vast Arctic seas.

After leaving Aklavik in September 1954, the Schaefers had returned to Edmonton and then set course for Germany, the country they would soon no longer call home. Their second son, Alfred, was born there on January 30, 1955. It was good to see friends and family again and to visit places like Otto's home town, Betzdorf. But Otto wanted to do more than socialize. He wanted to dig deeper into a field that really intrigued him: anthropology. "You must have a hobby," he said. "You cannot live to the full if you never go outside your profession."

While in Germany he spent many hours in libraries, learning all he could about the origins, physical characteristics, and culture of various racial groups. He had already recorded features and done measurements on the Inuit, including the size and shape of their skulls, average body height, and weight. In time to come, this "anthropometric" work, innocent as it seemed, would get him into a tight spot.

Crossing the Atlantic on the return journey, their small freighter ran into such a vicious storm, with "howling winds and mountainous waves," that they wondered if they really should be heading back to Canada at all. It took three weeks to reach Montreal.

Otto then headed for the Ottawa headquarters of the Department of Health and Welfare to spend a couple of weeks studying the files of patients from various parts of the Eastern Arctic. He spent another two weeks at Hamilton, home of the largest TB sanatorium in the British

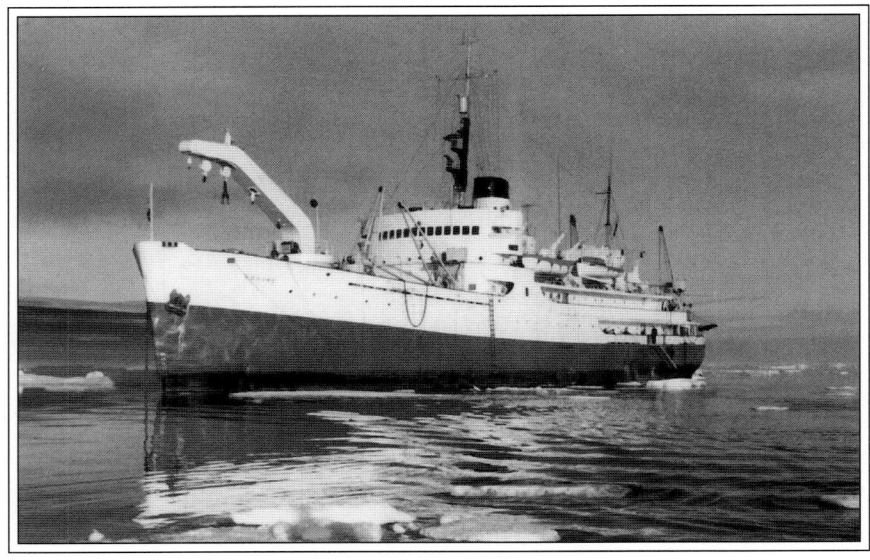

The Eastern Arctic Patrol ship C.D. Howe *near Resolute Bay in August 1955.*

Commonwealth, where specialists had been treating TB patients referred from the Eastern Arctic. There Otto learned current treatment methods and got experience in reading chest x-rays.

The *C.D. Howe* had been named after the flamboyant Minister of Trade and Commerce in the 1952 government of Prime Minister Louis St. Laurent. The ship was operated primarily by the Department of Transport, but the Departments of Health and Welfare and Northern Affairs also used its services. Over its long journey through northern waters, it would certainly run into channels and bays choked with ice. For such encounters, its bow was fitted with a sharp reinforcement that could chop through melting ice floes. But it could not cope with thick ice, which might block its path even in July. In that case, the captain might have to call in the stronger icebreaker *D'Iberville*, if it was in the vicinity, or simply change his route.

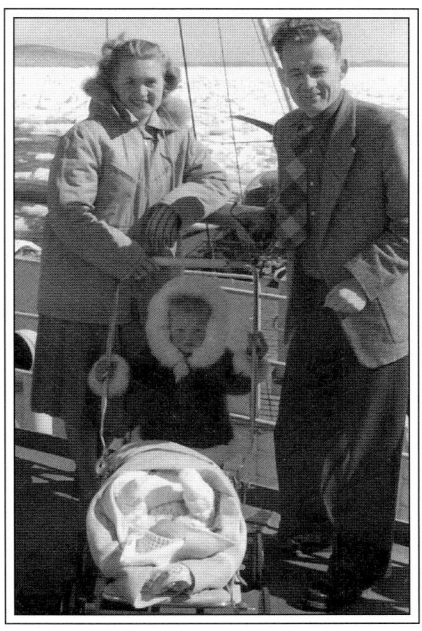

Didi and Otto Schaefer with their sons Lothar and Alfred on board the C.D. Howe *in August 1955.*

Besides large storage areas for freight and supplies, the *C.D. Howe* provided accommodation for Inuit patients being evacuated south for treatment or returning home. At the rear of the ship, outside the Schaefers' cabin, sat a helicopter on its landing pad. That helicopter got a lot of use. In the far North, it often took off to assess the extent of the ever-present enemy, sea ice, or to pick up or land returning patients if conditions did not permit a small boat or barge to be put ashore.

Little Lothar was fascinated to watch the great spinning propeller. He called the helicopter "Hoopie," a shortened version of *Hubschrauber*,

60 • Sunrise Over Pangnirtung

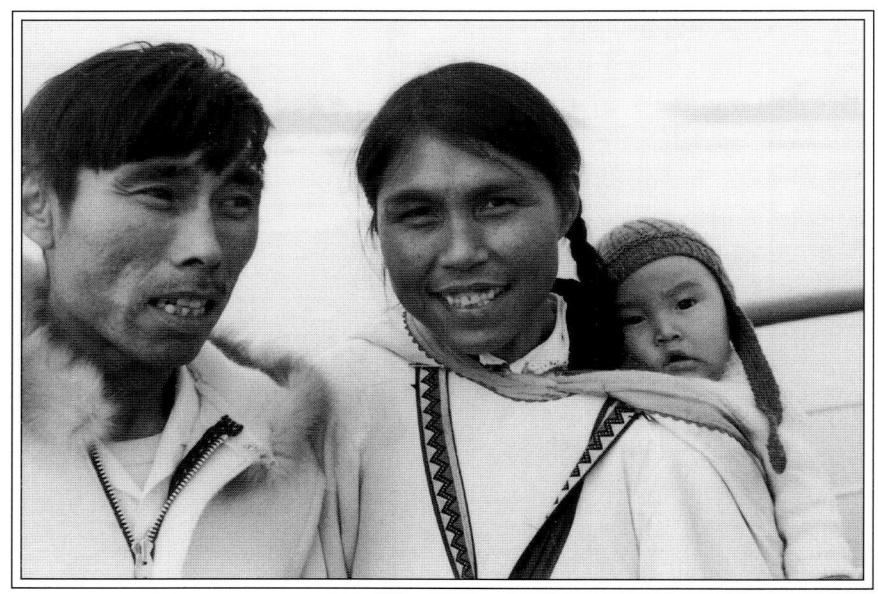

A family from Pond Inlet who were moving to Resolute Bay.

the German word for helicopter. He and the pilot became good friends. Lothar also had his own name for some people on board. Paulette Anerodluk, the young and much loved interpreter-cum-nursing aide from Coppermine, he called "Lett." Paulette had already spent years in hospital getting treatment for tuberculosis of her lungs and hip. Both her parents and nearly all her siblings had died of TB.

Otto's job at every port of call was to examine patients, x-ray their chests for TB, keep those needing evacuation on board, and inoculate children. Most patients came willingly to the ship, but some needed to be bribed: they would get tea and biscuits only after seeing the doctor. Otto found the medical facilities excellent, even good enough to allow him to do emergency surgery. One day he faced the prospect of having to do an operation on the *C.D. Howe*'s head nurse, Ann Webster. If he felt apprehensive, one can hardly blame him; operations on doctors and nurses are bound to go wrong. Ann was the daughter of the well-known and respected Reverend J. Harold Webster of Coppermine and Aklavik.

When she developed fever, vomiting, and pain in the lower abdomen, Otto diagnosed acute appendicitis, which usually requires prompt surgery. But operating on board ship was not without its hazards; both doctor and patient wondered if it would be safe to try some alternative treatment. Eventually they agreed to try antibiotics, an ice pack, liquid diet, and close observation, but it was risky.

Sleep did not come easily to Otto that night as doubts raced through his mind. Fortunately, the next day both fever and pain were subsiding. Ann continued to improve and eventually seemed well. But when the ship reached the port of Churchill, Otto sent her ashore—against her objections—to go south for surgery. He knew only too well that she might not be so fortunate if appendicitis struck again.

12
The Icy Waters of the Eastern Arctic

Even in late June, a fresh sea breeze from the northwest whistled across the deck of the *C.D. Howe* and brought out winter parkas. The ship was steering northward against the Labrador Stream that carried Arctic water and icebergs down from Greenland and Ellesmere Island in the high North.

Coming into Cape Hopes Advance on Ungava Bay, the captain saw the way blocked with jagged pressure ridges of pack ice. Again and again he drove the ship at full throttle, charging and ramming the icy barrier. The ship trembled and shook violently against the unyielding ice. Shaking his head, the captain decided to alter course, and headed across Hudson Strait for the south coast of Baffin Island.

At last Otto would catch a glimpse of that part of the world that had captured his boyhood imagination. On the map the ship's first destination, Lake Harbour (now Kimmirut), seemed tantalizingly near the beloved Cumberland Sound of his boyhood dreams. He looked longingly eastward, but realized that the *C.D. Howe* would need to blow a lot more black smoke from its funnels before those special bays and inlets came into view.

Why had Baffin Island so intrigued him? Canada's largest island (1500 km long) was hardly beautiful. In 1616, William Baffin had called it cruel, inhospitable, and lifeless. But he and other explorer-navigators before and after him were not looking for land. They were searching for the elusive Northwest Passage, and were prepared to risk life and limb to find it. Captain Thomas Button's fruitless 1612 expedition in the Hudson Bay area lost many men from malnutrition and disease (Neatby,

1958:32–33). But in 1616, Baffin chose a different course. He sailed up Davis Strait on the east coast of Baffin Island to a latitude of 73°N, where he reached Lancaster Sound. He looked west despairingly over "a bay choked with ice," gave up, and sailed back to England. Two centuries would pass before other explorers corrected the dreadful error he had made—the "bay choked with ice" was in reality the beginning of the Northwest Passage.

At Lake Harbour, site of Baffin Island's first Anglican Mission post (1909) and first Hudson Bay Company outpost (1911), a puny, three-month-old Inuk infant weighing less than 2.5 kg was brought on board for Otto to examine. Born with a harelip and cleft palate and therefore unable to suck, she was suffering from severe dehydration.

The baby's care became a Schaefer family affair. Six-month-old Alfred gave up his crib, Otto corrected the dehydration with infusions, and Didi carried on with hourly spoon feedings during the day. By the time the ship reached Fort Churchill two weeks later, the better-nourished baby was fit enough to be evacuated south for corrective surgery.

From Lake Harbour the *C.D. Howe* headed west to the settlement of Sugluk (Salluit) Inlet on the mainland. Originating from Sugluk, many of the most talented Inuit artists had travelled across Hudson Strait to Cape Dorset, where James Houston of the Montreal Arts Guild pioneered the growth and distribution of Inuit art.

No sooner had the ship dropped anchor near Sugluk than Otto got an urgent message to visit a group of very sick people about 20 km west of the settlement. One woman had coughed up a huge amount of blood. Otto flew by helicopter to the small settlement of half a dozen sealskin tents, and was most distressed to discover that almost one-third of the people he examined had active tuberculosis. Sugluk was almost as bad: 20 percent of the x-rays he took showed strong evidence of TB so severe that the patients had to be taken on board for eventual evacuation to the south. Otto felt depressed but gritted his teeth, more determined than ever to help rid the Inuit of this menace.

The *C.D. Howe* sailed west of the hamlet of Ivuyivik and entered the great watery expanse of Hudson Bay. As they travelled down the

64 • Sunrise Over Pangnirtung

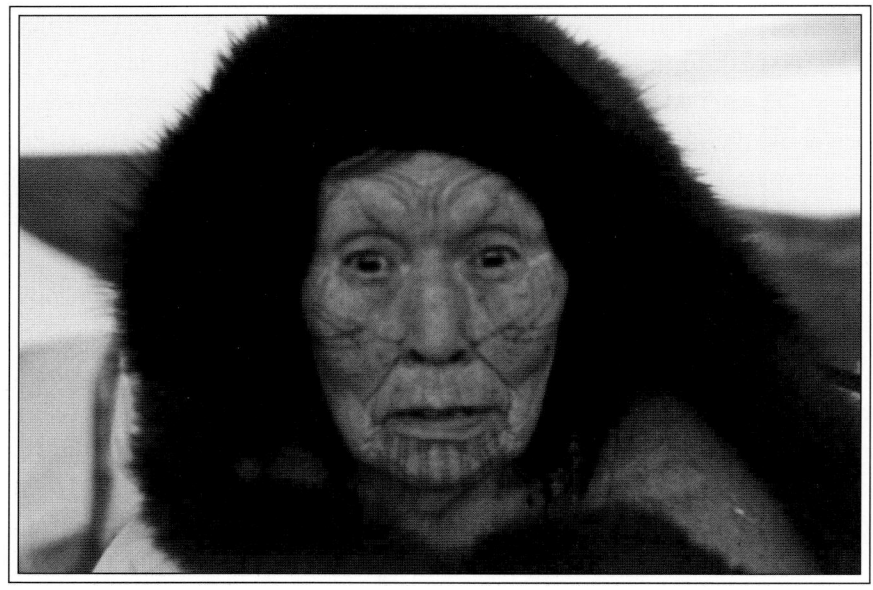

Supik, who was living at Craig Harbour in 1955.

featureless east coast, Otto thought that Henry Hudson and his mutinous crew must have followed a similar course in 1611 in the sailing ship *Discovery* (Neatby, 1958). The rebellious crew had forced Captain Hudson and a handful of loyal crew members into a boat without food, water, or oars and cut her loose. Then the *Discovery* sailed off, leaving Hudson and his companions to drift helplessly. Otto had seen a painting of the cluster of doomed men huddled together in a small boat. The painting was not entirely imaginary—Abacuck Prickett, a "neutral" member of Hudson's crew, had kept a detailed diary of the entire tragic ordeal.

A few days later, after depositing the sick baby and about 20 patients with advanced TB at Fort Churchill, Otto looked out of his cabin/examining room and rubbed his eyes in disbelief. It looked as though the ghosts of Henry Hudson and his condemned men were still drifting. A motorboat with seven waving Inuit aboard floated motionless on the waves. They had left on a small seal-hunting trip two days before, only

The Icy Waters of the Eastern Arctic • 65

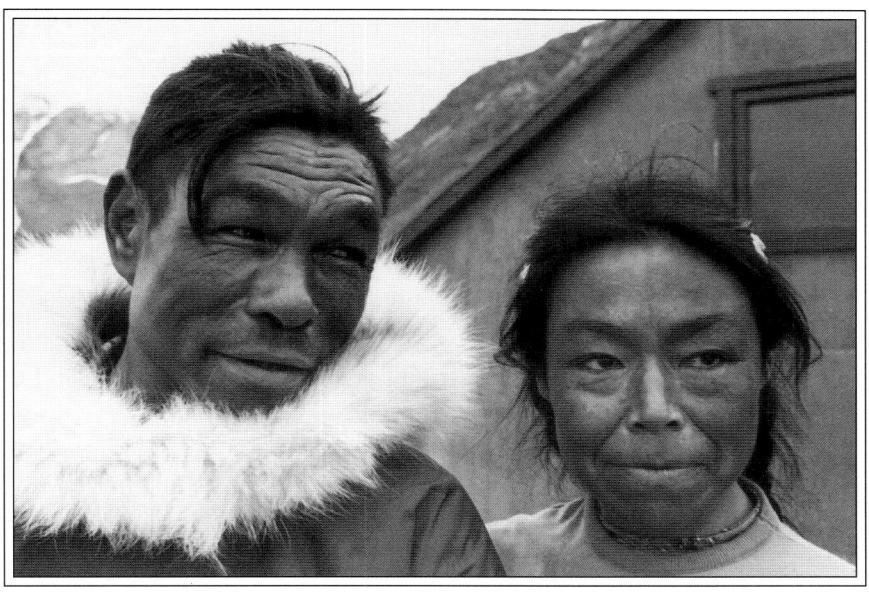

Mosesie, a well-known carver from Inukjuak on the east coast of Hudson Bay, and his wife. Mosesie carved a hunter and a harpooned walrus for Otto.

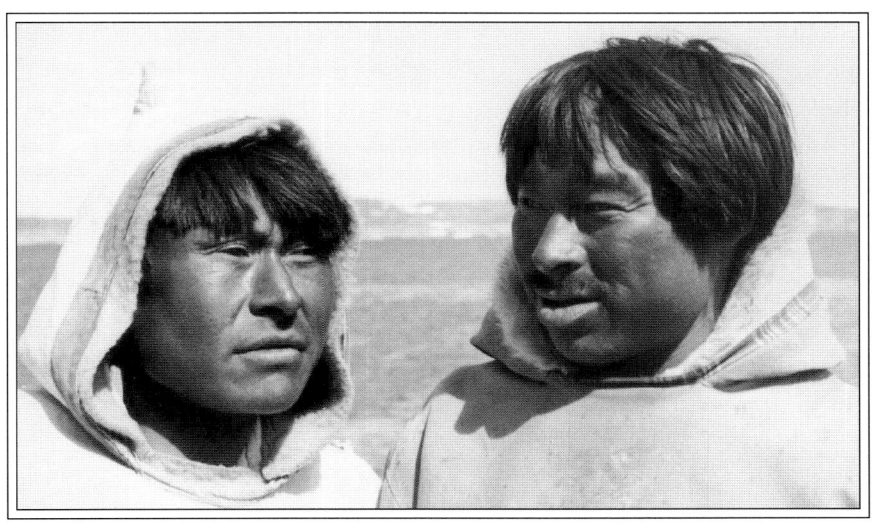

Inuit from the Cape Dorset area.

to lose their propeller. Without food and at the mercy of an adverse wind that blew them farther and farther from home, they had drifted as helplessly as the victims of the 1611 mutiny. These drifters, however, were quickly rescued with the captain's motorboat, and their own boat was winched on board. Then they were given hot tea and some food before being taken to Coral Harbour on Southampton Island, one of the main airports and supply points of the DEW line. Otto wondered: is it possible that Henry Hudson's men could also have been rescued?

The physical features of the Inuit continued to intrigue him. In Lake Harbour, he saw a conspicuous admixture of "white" blood, probably from Scottish and American whalers two generations before. The Inuit of Arctic Quebec, especially the Ungava Bay area, did not show the mongoloid features that he had noticed around Aklavik. On Baffin Island, the heads he measured were more oblong than rounded, in contrast to those in the Mackenzie Delta. Apparently the inhabitants of the Arctic came from several diverse "streams." Yet despite this ethnological diversity, they spoke a common language—with minor differences in dialect—that could be understood from the Chukotsk Peninsula of Siberia to eastern Greenland.

From Coral Harbour they steamed east along the length of Hudson Strait, cruising along easily, riding one of the highest tides in the world. In 1578, on his third and last expedition, Martin Frobisher had encountered a "powerful current of tide" that impeded progress as he tried to sail into Hudson Strait (Neatby, 1958:4).

13
Baffin Island

On July 30, 1955, as the *C.D. Howe* rounded Resolution Island at the southern tip of Baffin Island, Otto felt he was getting close to the land of his hero, Franz Boas. But before the ship could drop anchor, he got a message calling him to see a sick boy on the island. He took off immediately in the helicopter. The weak, feverish and almost unconscious child was probably suffering from tuberculous meningitis. Otto took the child back to the ship and started treatment right away, after doing a spinal tap to confirm the diagnosis. The child appeared to be getting better before his evacuation to the south for institutional care.

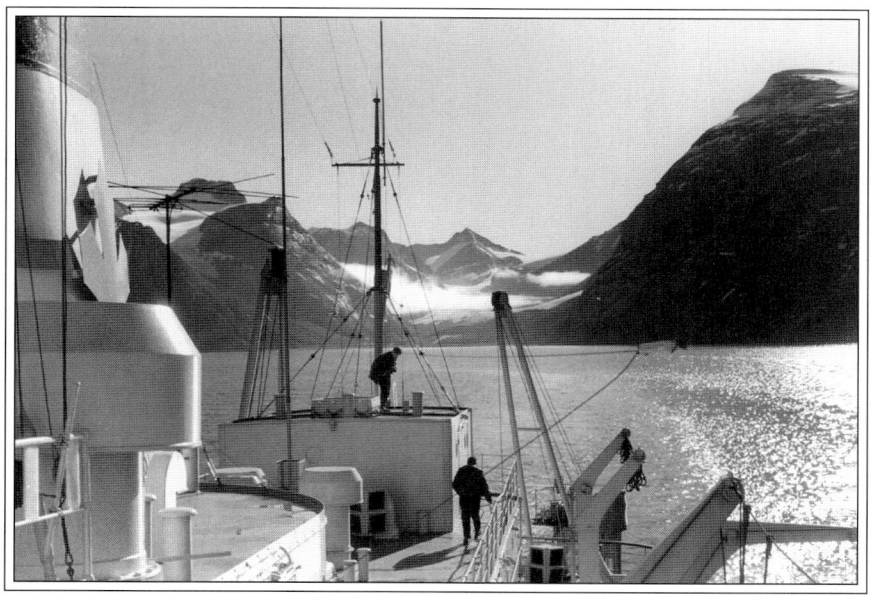

The C.D. Howe *sailing in Inugsuin Fiord, south of Clyde River.*

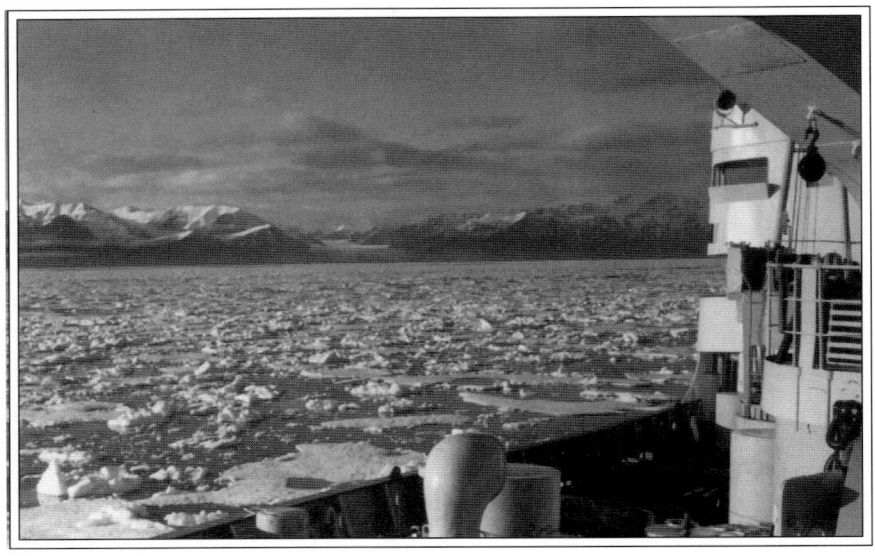

View from Pond Inlet north to Bylot Island, as seen from the C.D. Howe.

The ship cruised past the entrance to Cumberland Sound that night and headed up the east coast of Baffin Island the next day. On the left rose the great mountains and granite cliffs of the Cumberland Peninsula. Masses of pack ice clung to the foot of the cliffs. The ship picked its way slowly northwestward through bands of ice floes and small icebergs. Surrounded by snow, sleet, and fog, the passengers felt they were traversing a ghostly world. But the next day, clear and breezeless, brought its own equally weird and unnatural phenomenon—the fata morgana, with its mirror-images of islands and icebergs above the horizon, like the mirages of the Sahara desert.

Stopping at Pond Inlet and Arctic Bay at the north end of Baffin Island, Otto got some good news: the Inuit were definitely healthier and suffered less from tuberculosis than those from any other settlement. He thought that the presence of more fish and sea mammals in their diet made for better nutrition and therefore stronger resistance to disease.

To get to Arctic Bay, they had passed by Bylot Island, with its mighty icecap and tumbling glaciers. Who was Robert Bylot? A controversial figure, he had stood by in 1611, not playing a direct part in the sordid plot that set Henry Hudson adrift to die. But a month later, when several of the mutineers were killed by angry Inuit near Digges Island at the entrance to Hudson Bay, he alone possessed the navigational skill to guide the *Discovery* back to England. With Bylot at the helm, the ship eventually reached home safely. Instead of getting the hangman's noose, the usual punishment for mutineers, Bylot was pardoned and vindicated. He subsequently joined William Baffin for his next expedition (Neatby, 1958:34).

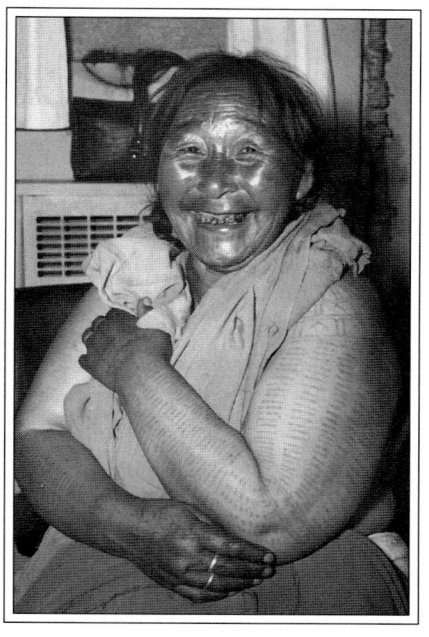

Attuat from Arctic Bay.

At Arctic Bay, Otto saw several not-so-young ladies with intricate tattoos of face, arms, and torso. He managed to get a picture of Attuat, whom he described as "somewhat domineering, a strong voice in her community, and on her fourth husband." Many years later, when introduced to Pierre Trudeau, Attuat would give the prime minister a bear hug that left him gasping for breath.

On August 10, after ploughing the way through fields of pack ice in Lancaster Sound, the *C.D. Howe* reached Resolute Bay on Cornwallis Island, just below 75°N. Originally a weather station for the Canadian Arctic Archipelago, Resolute had grown in size and importance during the Cold War with the establishment of an airport. Five Inuit families disembarked here, having accepted the invitation from the federal government to move from their homes on the east shore of Hudson Bay, where the seal population was becoming depleted.

At Resolute Bay, the local RCMP constable approached Otto, asking for medical help for a woman in labour. Her two previous deliveries

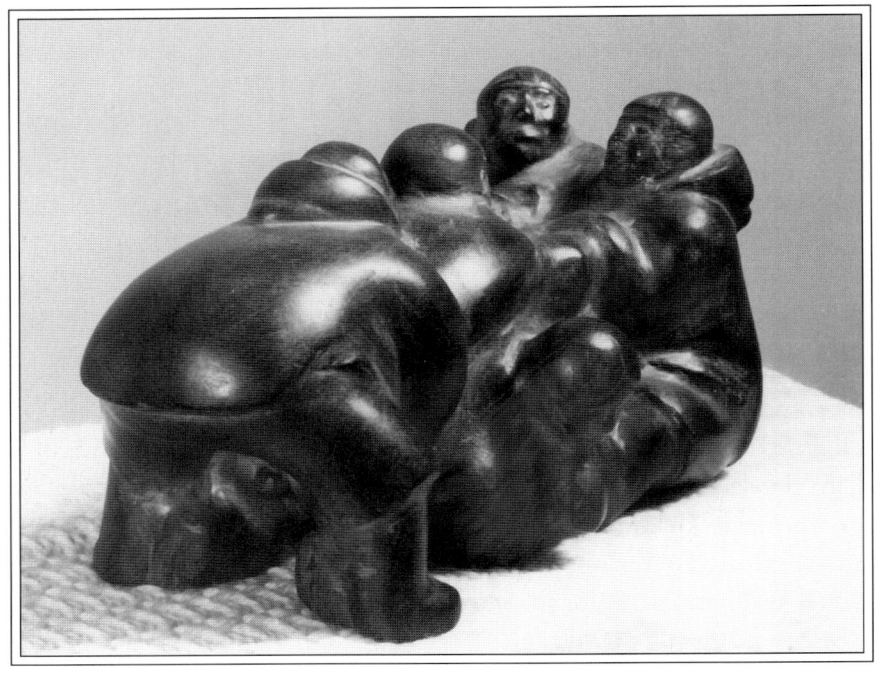

Soapstone carving of childbirth made by Makpa from Baker Lake.

had been prolonged and complicated. Otto went along, planning not to interfere but to help the midwife (mother from the tent next door) if need be. He wrote in his journal:

> *The expectant mother was kneeling on a caribou skin, with her elbows resting on a footstool. Her husband tried to comfort her by pressing with both hands down on her back, while two young men pulled on her arms and shoulders. When the baby's head started crowning, she reclined on to her back, and the two young men pressed the side of her womb while her husband pushed on the fundus [upper part]. As soon as the baby started crying, it was handed to the mother.... . After about half an hour, I thought it was time to feel the uterus and attempt to push the placenta out. That idea was met, however, with strong opposition from mother, midwife, and husband. The mother*

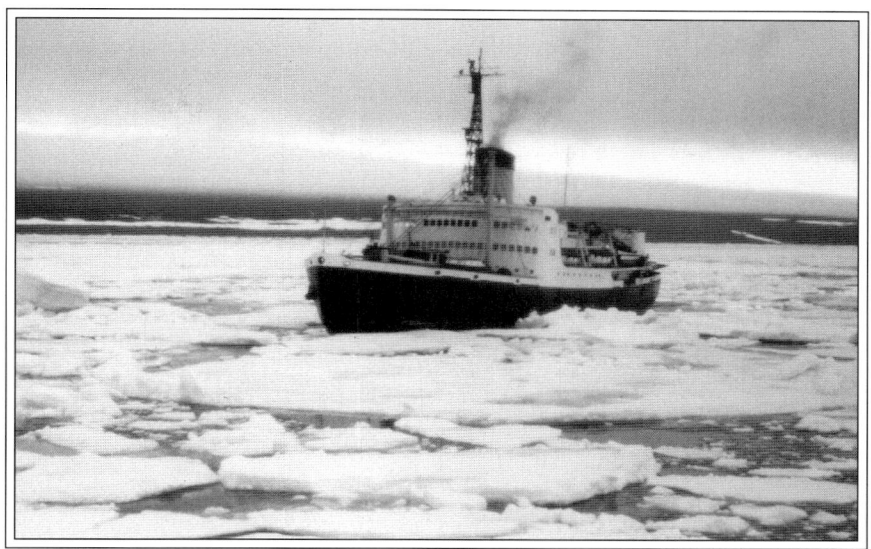

The icebreaker D'Iberville *in Lancaster Sound.*

got up on her knees again, and in no time the placenta landed on the caribou skin. The blood-stained caribou skin with placenta was carried out to the dogs and a new skin placed under her.... I had to admit that they had remarkably good ideas and practices suiting their living conditions.

On August 20, the *C.D. Howe* found itself completely walled in by old, firm polar ice floes and thick pack ice. To the rescue came the *D'Iberville*, Canada's largest icebreaker, which happened to be in the vicinity. With black smoke belching from its stacks, it attacked: charging, riding up and over, and crunching the underlying ice. The icebreaker cleared a narrow but adequate channel, and the *C.D. Howe* steamed off towards Grise Fiord on Ellesmere Island, the most northerly of Canada's islands. But rounding the east coast of Devon Island, with its 2000 metre ice-capped mountains, they found the bay before Grise Fiord clogged with ice floes. They dropped anchor and waited. Fortunately, during the night a strong northerly wind broke up and cleared much of the ice, so that the ship's barges could approach the shore to bring people on board for examination.

For the Schaefer family, the long journey by ship was coming to an end. Dodging icebergs and ice floes, the *C.D. Howe* turned south, retracing its course down the east coast of Baffin Island. On September 9, 1955, they reached the beautiful natural harbour of Padloping, on the other side of the mountains from Pangnirtung, and Otto knew he was not far from "home."

That night the captain and crew held a farewell party on board ship for the Schaefer family, who had endeared themselves to all. The ship's chef presented them with a stuffed turkey, a ham, and a special farewell cake. The medical team, consisting of another doctor, two nurses, and Paulette Anerodluk, gave them a beautiful soapstone carving of a hunter paddling his kayak.

Next morning, on a clear, sunny day, the ship turned into Cumberland Sound and steamed towards Pangnirtung Fiord, with its lacy network of creeks and waterfalls. This was the place that had entranced Franz Boas back in 1883. On the right soared rugged cliffs and mountains surmounted by the sparkling, massive whiteness of the

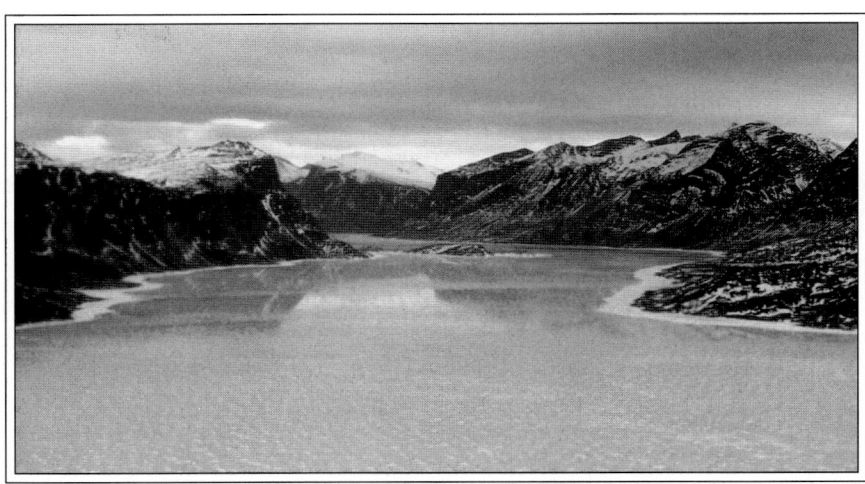

Upper Pangnirtung Fiord.

Penny Ice Cap, which now crowns the heights of Auyuittuq National Park. It seemed as if the mighty forces of nature had conspired to welcome them.

Waving good-bye to their shipboard friends, Otto and Didi boarded the ship's barge with their two boys and possessions to last for the next two years. The *C.D. Howe* departed the next day on its return trip to Montreal, leaving the little family to make a new home in Pangnirtung, "the place of the bull caribou"(Harper, 1997:303).

14
Early Days in Pangnirtung

BRITISH explorer John Davis, boyhood friend of Sir Walter Raleigh, may have been the first European to enter Cumberland Sound, in 1585. He had been heading north up Davis Strait (named after him) in his 50-ton sailing ship, the *Sunshine*, believing that the top of the globe was "an ice-free space" that would allow clear passage to the Orient. When bad weather drove him back, Davis rounded the Cumberland Peninsula on the southern end of Baffin Island and turned into Cumberland Sound. He described the coastline as "barren without woods or grass, the rocks faire like marble, full of vaines of diverse colours" (Neatby, 1958:8). Deeply recessed with bays and inlets, Cumberland Sound is 300 km long, with an average width of 65 km. The hamlet of Pangnirtung sits on a narrow coastal plain on the eastern shore of Pangnirtung Fiord. The Pangnirtung Pass of lakes, waterfalls and glaciers leads up to spectacular Auyuittuq ("the land that never melts") National Park, established in 1972 as Canada's first national park reserve north of the Arctic Circle (Rigby, 1997:296). In August 1999, Auyuittuq was officially elevated from a national park reserve to a national park.

The newly arrived family had known what to expect, but the towering cliffs and steep-sided fjords and mountains almost overwhelmed them. As Didi commented, it was beauty and grandeur on a scale they had never imagined. Emmi Nemetz, one of the nurses, echoed her words: "I had never seen such splendour in my whole life. And the stillness and the mystery were cathedral-like. Later I realized it really was God's great cathedral."

In the small community at Pangnirtung, along with the Inuit residents lived 17 white people who worked for the mission hospital, the RCMP, and the Hudson's Bay Company store. Around the perimeter of

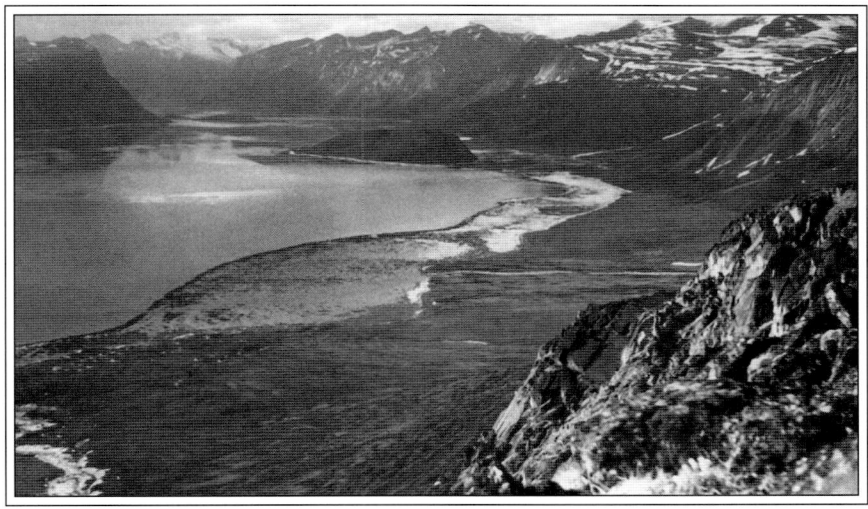

A view of upper Pangnirtung Fiord, with the settlement on the lower left.

Cumberland Sound lived about 600 Inuit, mostly in camps. It would be Otto's responsibility to visit each of these 14 camps twice a year, as well as 3 others over the mountains on Davis Strait. During the two-month period after spring breakup, some of the camps could be reached by boat. Otherwise he would have to rely on his dog team, taking medicines and supplies along with him in a big box. The noisy but speedy snowmobile had not yet arrived on the scene.

The 20-bed St. Luke's Anglican Hospital, health care centre for some 800 Inuit and white people scattered across the region, had started in a small way in 1928 (Brett, 1969). The original one-room shack had space for seven patients, but once during an epidemic 38 desperately sick people had been jammed in. Even after subsequent expansion, it still overflowed at times. Then Otto had to find mattresses and stretchers to lay in the hall and even in the attic, where the lab and his tiny office were located.

Dr. Leslie Livingstone had signed on in 1922 as the first resident doctor to the Inuit. After making several annual trips to the Eastern Arctic as the ship's doctor on board the S.S. *Arctic* in 1923–25, he took up residence at Pangnirtung in 1926. The first physician to work in the new hospital, Dr. Livingstone also built the doctor's little house in 1931. Etuangat, the doctor's helper and interpreter, assisted with the building along with his other jobs. Otto would soon get to know this remarkable man.

Life was much more primitive at Pangnirtung than it had been at Aklavik. For one thing, people had to carry drinking water in a sled-tank from a river that flowed into the saltwater fjord. After freeze-up, splintered ice was brought from the river and melted for drinking. The hospital kept one barrel of drinking water and two of melted snow for other uses. Surgical instruments were boiled or sterilized in a pressure cooker. Electricity came from two small generators: one for the hospital and one for the police post. The Schaefers got by with oil lamps for most of a year until a generator arrived for their house.

The sole source of heat for the Schaefer house was a coal-burning cookstove that also melted snow in its reservoir. A nearby barrel held melted river ice for drinking. Otto stoked the stove before going to bed and set his alarm to feed it again at 3:00 a.m. Fortunately they had brought warm eiderdown comforters and pyjamas for themselves and the children. But the floor, with its multiple holes and crevices, was so cold that Didi nearly always wore her felt boots. Behind the stove was the "sitting room," with just enough space for a sofa. Next to it was a stand for the Schaefers' radio/record player from Germany. A mobile ladder

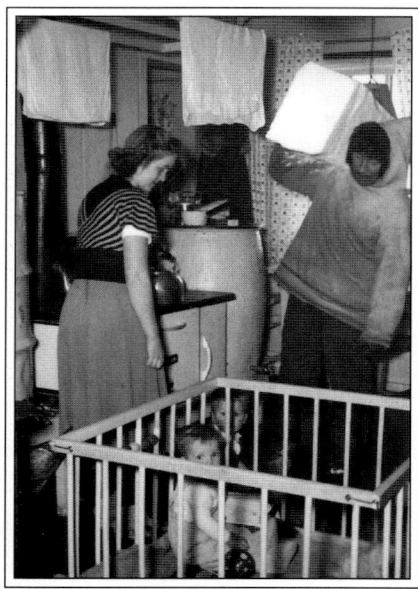

Etuangat bringing in a block of snow to be melted in a barrel beside the kitchen stove in the Schaefers' house.

allowed access to the small attic, where they stored special treats like fresh food. Otto's desk somehow found a place in the small kitchen, though his chair backed onto the icewater barrel. Empty cardboard boxes served as his filing cabinets. Simple activities like having a sort of bath and using the toilet provided challenges for the whole family.

Once a year the Hudson's Bay Company ship S.S. *Rupertsland* brought in a year's supply of groceries and other needs. But everything—meat, fish, vegetables, and fruit—came in cans. They soon tired of opening tins and found themselves relishing the local food of seal and caribou meat and fish. No one had any success with a garden—the rocky soil with permafrost a couple of inches beneath it, combined with a short growing season and bitter winds, put a stop to that.

In Otto and Didi's little house, the warmth, cheer, and hospitality seemed to sweep aside the drabness and starkness. As nurse Norma Westgate remembered, "A lot of things happened there and we had

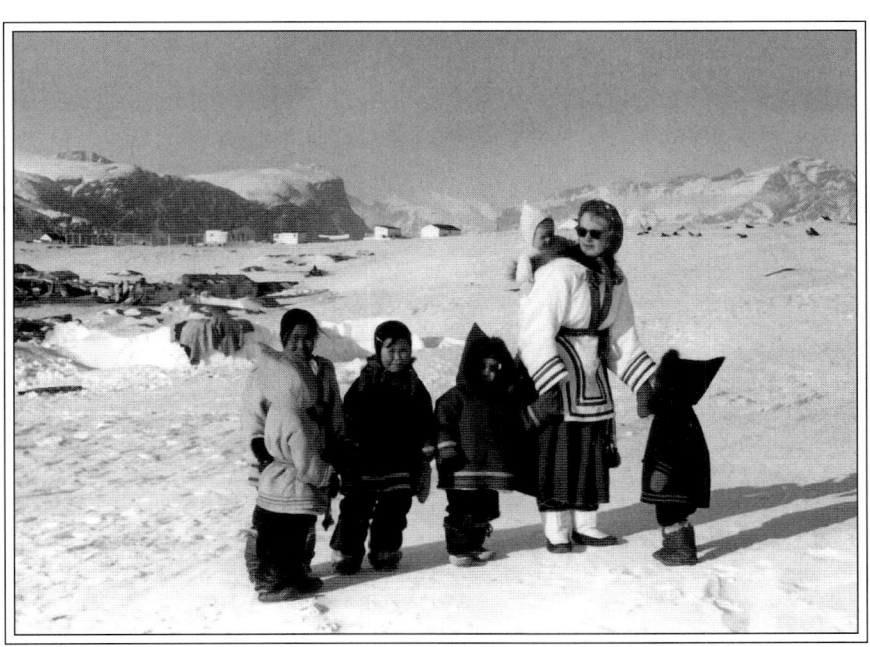

Didi with her sons and Inuit children in April 1957.

many happy, joyful times. Christmas especially was wonderful with lots of family customs like candles on the tree."

Two months after arriving, Otto received a letter of invitation from an old friend and colleague in family practice near Nelson, British Columbia: Would Otto consider leaving "the desolate, dark Arctic" next summer to join him? Otto found it easy to decline. "Didi and I feel like we're living in a veritable paradise," he replied. "We are too happy here to even think about leaving."

15
Etuangat

It was almost daybreak. The hamlet of Pangnirtung still lay bathed in the long shadows of the mountains. But outside the little hospital, impatient dogs yelped in their harness and a few people scurried about in the grey light of dawn. Otto Schaefer and his Inuit helper and guide, Etuangat, were busy preparing for a four-week trip by dogsled to camps over the mountains on Davis Strait. They had loaded the long *komatik*, sled, with medicines, food, warm clothes—everything they might possibly need for the long trip. Otto was getting anxious and just a bit irritable. He had desperately wanted to be away well before dawn. He watched while Joapie, Etuangat's five-year-old adopted son, tried hard to tighten the ropes lashing the load to the *komatik*. The boy tugged and strained hard, but the load was far from firm. It just wasn't good enough, and Otto pushed him aside.

Then they were on their way. But it wasn't such a good day. Usually Otto and Etuangat chatted and joked, mostly in Inuktitut. But Etuangat remained sullen and silent. The next day Otto got annoyed and said so, but no reply came. The third day was hard going; the dogs strained to drag the sled over the rough, rocky terrain and skimpy snow cover. They stopped to rest and brew tea. Sitting with a cup of tea in his hand, Etuangat finally spoke:

Doc, I somehow thought that you understood us Inuit better than the other kadluna *(white people). But just before we left, I saw you push Joapie out of the way, acting no better than the rest of them. Maybe you didn't see that I waited until he was a bit away from me before I re-tightened the ropes. Our boys learn by doing the same as we do and we don't push them away; we don't*

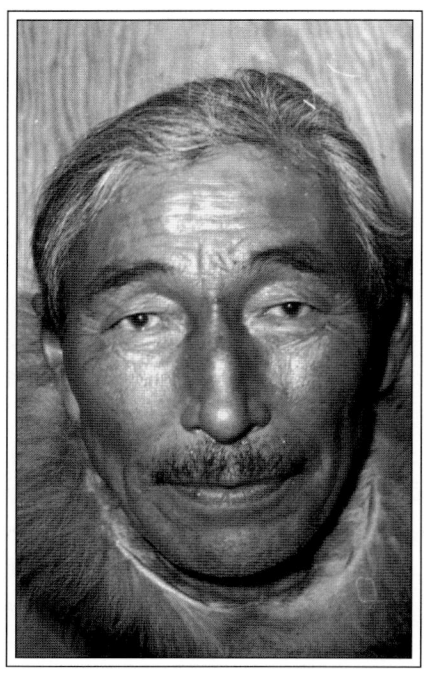

Etuangat in 1957.

even let them see or feel if their work has to be redone; they help better when you make them feel they are needed and useful. Joapie will not try to help us for a long time to come, now that you have pushed him away as useless.

He had spoken softly, almost inaudibly, but Otto received the message very clearly. He felt chastened by it, and was determined to learn from it. He would learn other lessons too from his middle-aged Inuit helper as they travelled, built snow houses, and ate chunks of half-frozen caribou together.

Gentle but down-to-earth, Etuangat had a few other ideas—sound, if a bit harsh—about preparing children for the realities of the world. When they were on a journey, they usually slept in their canvas tent and put a polar bear skin down on the ground with a caribou hide on top, hair up. On this warm protective cover, they laid their sleeping bags.

On one trip Etuangat's 17-year-old son Amosie came along. Otto was surprised to see that the boy rated only a thin piece of worn caribou skin to lie on the cold ground.

"There's not much fur left on that piece of hide," he told Etuangat.

"Maybe so," he answered. "But we have to educate our sons, or they'll never get used to the cold. That little strip of caribou skin will do the job. We can't afford to spoil our sons or our dogs."

Born at a place south of Broughton Island on Davis Strait, Etuangat was a little unsure of his age but said he could remember seeing a baby—

known to have been born in 1903—carried in his mother's parka. That memory would put his date of birth around the beginning of the century. He credited his survival to the fact that right after his birth an *angakok* (medicine man) had shouted "mighty words into my ears." His mother had lost nearly all her previous children in infancy.

Etuangat had known hardship and personal tragedy. His wife had died suddenly as a young woman, leaving him with three small children to care for. He had desperately needed someone to be their mother. When the Reverend John Turner told him about Nukinga, who was 15 years older than he was, Etuangat was surprised. Then he realized that what he really wanted was a woman experienced in caring for children. Nukinga proved to be a wise choice.

A few years earlier, Etuangat and his older brother had been out caribou hunting. They separated, in the hopes of driving the animals into each other's rifle range. Suddenly a blizzard struck. With the blizzard still raging, Etuangat waited for two more days before going to a settlement about 80 km away for help. But he never saw his brother again. Young hunters often disappeared that way, he said. He told the story without any display of emotion, concluding with the word symbolizing Inuit philosophy: *Ayunamat* (it can't be helped).

Otto was still struggling to improve his English when confronted with the reason and motivation to learn another language. "In my country, you speak Inuktitut," Etuangat had said. Otto was willing to give it a try, but needed help. "Will you come to my house every evening and start my immersion course?" he asked. Etuangat did just that, taking Didi into the class too. Not surprisingly, Didi's skills soon surpassed her husband's.

Otto denies that he ever gained much fluency, but others have said he seemed to be at home in the language. Dr. Maurice Beare, Otto's associate at the Charles Camsell Hospital, claimed that Otto was the only physician to learn Inuktitut. Otto denies that claim, however, saying Dr. Jim Osborne of Vancouver and Dr. B. Sabean, who succeeded him in Pangnirtung, were both fluent in the language. In Aklavik most people spoke English, but in Pangnirtung the main language was Inuktitut.

His knowledge of their native language would strengthen Otto's relationship with the Inuit.

Etuangat also made it clear that it was time to put away the disparaging label *Eskimo* (Eaters of raw meat), used first by Indians and later by Europeans. His people liked to be called *Inuit* (the People). An individual should be called an *Inuk*.

Otto learned to rely heavily on Etuangat's judgement, acquired during years of guiding and helping the resident doctors, beginning with Dr. Livingstone. He trusted his knowledge of patients, their families, and their medical histories more than any hospital or resident doctor's files.

With time their friendship grew, and they worked together as equals. Taoya, Otto and Didi's daughter, was born at Pangnirtung and of course has no memory of Etuangat. But in later years she had learned enough to be able to say, "There are few people on this earth that my dad respects more than Etuangat."

16
The Hard Life

IN 1883, Franz Boas had been deeply moved by the incredible physical endurance, courage and fortitude, and resourcefulness of the Inuit. He was sent to study their country, but they became his friends. Seventy-five years later, Otto Schaefer was no less impressed.

One day in November, a team of dogs hauled in a man with a broken femur. He had fallen on a sharp rock while fishing in a freshwater lake only 60 km from Pangnirtung on the other side of Cumberland Sound. On good solid sea ice, his rescuers could have reached the hospital in less than two days. Sadly, a storm with strong winds had broken up much of the new sea ice. Standing on the shore, they were faced with only treacherous ice floes and open water. They had no choice but to take the long, rough trip inland, climbing over a series of steep moraines and hills to reach a valley that led down to Pangnirtung Fiord. Every minute of the seven-day journey jolting over the barren rocky hills and valleys with little or no snow cover must have been agonizing for the injured man. No one had anything to give him for pain.

No plane or helicopter could land at Pangnirtung under the prevailing conditions—Otto would have to care for the patient himself. An x-ray showed the fracture to be a bad one, with much separation of the broken fragments. First Otto gave the stalwart patient a light anaesthetic. Then, to restore the thigh bone to its normal alignment, he got two strong Inuit men to pull on his shoulders and two others to pull his lower leg in the opposite direction. While the four men were straining at their job, he applied a large plaster cast. He had hoped to take another x-ray to check the position of the broken bone, but unfortunately the hospital's generator failed.

Not until mid-January was the ice on the Sound solid enough (as determined by the local RCMP officer) for a DC 3 from Labrador to land. The plane brought in a new generator and took Otto's patient down to Montreal. Several weeks later the word came back: the orthopaedic surgeons in Montreal reported that the treatment given in Pangnirtung was adequate. Nothing further had to be done.

The other passenger on that southbound DC 3 was Tapitia, a young woman referred south for treatment of tuberculosis and "psychological assessment." Tapitia was the sole survivor of the 1937–38 famine that had taken the lives of all 40 residents of an Inuit camp in the Cape Dyer area, on the east coast of Cumberland Peninsula. Huge quantities of heavy, soft snow had fallen. Dogs could not run in it, and hunters found it impossible to move. After food supplies dwindled, they ate their dogs until not one was left. One man set out on his own, struggling to reach his brother's camp. He died a few kilometres away. In his pocket was a note in syllabic symbols (the written form of Inuktitut) describing the monstrous snowfall that had doomed them all. At the time Tapitia had been with relatives living in a camp south of Cape Dyer. Her life had been spared, but she was miserable, jostled around from one set of relatives to another. Otto was less concerned over her physical state than with her disturbed personality. Like others who have been neglected and abused as children, she needed counselling and support before returning to Pangnirtung.

One man with severe frostbite symbolized not just the harshness of the North, but the toughness and courage of its people. Early in December, when the temperature hovered around -35°C, Amosie and Paulusie, Etuangat's son and son-in-law, brought in Ahmi, a 19-year-old man in critical condition. Three days before, Ahmi had been seal hunting with other men on the sea ice near the northwestern coast of Cumberland Sound. Before they knew what was happening, a gale-force wind had ripped off the ice floe on which they were standing. Most of the men scrambled back to the safety of the land-fast ice. But young Ahmi, with his dogs, a loaded *komatik*, and an older man, Auyalo, drifted on the floating ice towards the east side of the Sound, where they came to a band of thin, broken-off shore ice.

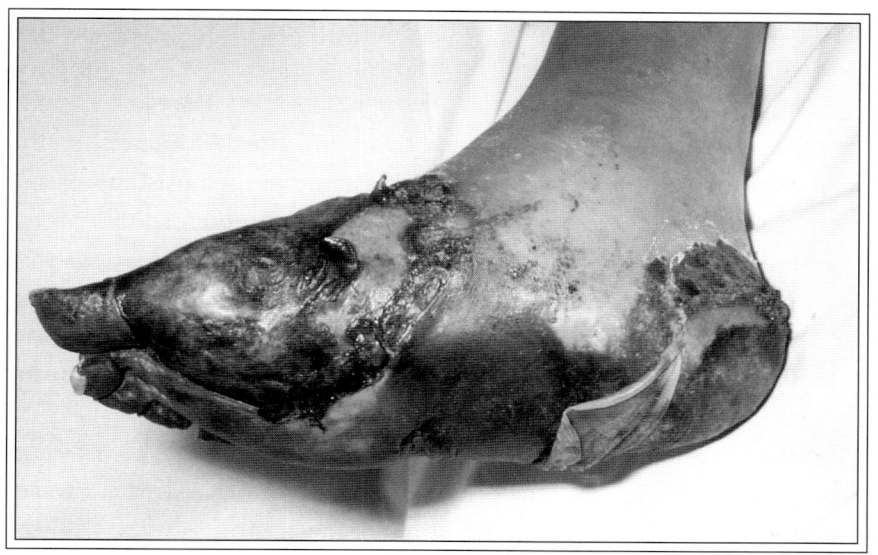

A severely frostbitten foot. Photo by Gerald Hankins.

Auyalo probed the thin ice with his harpoon rod. Ahmi was supposed to follow behind at a safe distance, but suddenly his dogs raced for the shore. The ice broke under the weight of the loaded sled, and Ahmi was thrown into the frigid water. He pulled himself partly out by grabbing the dogs' harness and finally got onto firm ice.

They looked for snow for Ahmi to roll himself in, but there was none. Then they ran a few kilometres along the shore, until they found enough snow. Working desperately against time, Auyalo built a makeshift igloo and lit his primus stove. Ahmi wisely kept running in circles but eventually fell exhausted to the ground. Auyalo hauled the young man into the igloo. With the primus, he tried to thaw Ahmi's boots, now filled with rock-hard ice. Ahmi no longer felt any pain. The heat of the little stove slowly thawed his frozen boots. Then Auyalo pulled them off and tried to thaw Ahmi's frozen feet by rubbing them inside his own fur clothing.

After an hour, the kerosene ran out. Without dry clothes, sleeping bags, or food (they had been hunting close to their home camp), chances of survival seemed nil. But Auyalo refused to quit and constantly goaded his companion to keep moving around, waving his arms, stamping the snow, anything.

When the blizzard subsided the second morning, Auyalo lashed the listless young man on his sled and raced his dogs to the next Inuit camp. From there, a new team rushed them to Pangnirtung Hospital.

Ahmi developed dry gangrene of both feet, but Otto thought that given the circumstances, the outcome could have been much worse. In time it became clear that Ahmi would lose half of his right foot and the two small toes on his left foot. Otto sent him south by plane two months after the accident.

Auyalo himself did not come to the hospital. If he had, Otto—and undoubtedly others too—would certainly have offered him a warm handshake. As it was, the people of his home camp rewarded him for his noble, life-saving efforts by making him camp boss!

17
Folk Lore and Ingenuity

LIVING in isolation and without access to any kind of medical care before the arrival of mission hospitals and nursing stations, Inuit scattered across the northern barrens had devised their own remedies. Some "cures" and treatments were based on sound observation and logic; others were not quite so sound. Otto freely admitted that he came to the North with a "haughty disregard" for any kind of folk medicine. Later, instead of ridiculing traditional beliefs and practices, he tried to understand them. In many cases, he gained a real appreciation.

On one occasion while visiting a hunting camp on Cumberland Sound far from Pangnirtung, he was astounded to see a little girl with a fine, hairline scar about four inches long across her forehead. The child's mother explained that several months previously, she had slipped and cut her head on the sharp edge of a broken ice-slab. Like all scalp wounds, the deep gash bled profusely. With no hope for treatment elsewhere, the ingenious mother determined to do the job herself. She cut a long sheath of her daughter's thick, black hair and threaded it through her fur-sewing needle. Then she proceeded to sew up the gaping wound. It looked like the work of a plastic surgeon, Otto thought, assuring the mother that even in sterile hospital conditions, he could not have done a finer job.

Otto had read about the resourceful Indian woman who repaired the broken kneecap of a man by using a suture of caribou sinew to hold the fragments together. For anaesthesia, she gave the patient "a fairly hot coal" to hold in his hand, as a sort of counter-irritant.

Some traditional techniques were inappropriate, or even harmful. Otto took a picture of one man whose *angakok* uncle had made several cuts to "let the water out" of his swollen knee joint. No water drained out and—fortunately—no infection got into the joint. But that same *angakok* had done textbook surgery a few years before when he made a cut over a man's distended bladder. When urine gushed forth, the sudden relief of great pain was dramatic.

One young man even made his own dentures. The teeth in his upper jaw gradually decayed, probably because of his liking for sweet foods from the Hudson's Bay Company store. Some fell out, and others were extracted by the ship's dentist on the annual visit. With nothing but gums left, he proceeded to make his own denture out of ivory from a walrus tusk. Seeing this handiwork, Otto's own jaw dropped in amazement: the man had achieved what dentists call "perfect occlusion." The new denture fitted so well that he could even chew *muktuk* (whale skin).

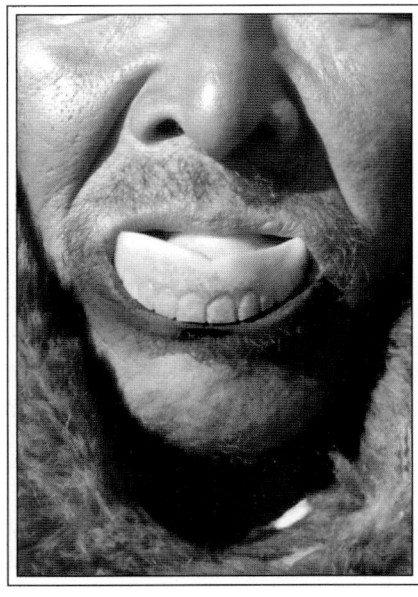

Otoki from Cape Dorset, showing the dentures that he carved for himself from walrus ivory.

Undoubtedly one of the most colourful "caregivers" around Cumberland Sound was old Ashevaq from Illongaya settlement. Half-white, she claimed that her father was a sea captain. She was at least 75, and rheumatoid arthritis had seriously deformed her hands. Ashevaq had acquired a reputation—likely justified—as a skillful remover of placentas retained after childbirth. She had probably saved the lives of many young women. Otto came across the weather-beaten old veteran while visiting Illongaya camp one day. Looking at her knobbly fingers and grubby, long fingernails, he asked her what she did before inserting her hands into the wombs of women who had just had a baby.

"You think I don't know what to do?" she asked. "I just chew down the ends of my fingernails and go ahead with the job."

For some Inuit, the prospect of having to be evacuated to Montreal or Hamilton for treatment of tuberculosis was intolerable, even though the treatment was free. The disruption was more than they could bear, and they thought it would be better to die. Older people sometimes chose to take their own lives, rather than be a burden to their families. Otto knew of several elderly Inuit who had quietly walked out into the winter night to freeze to death.

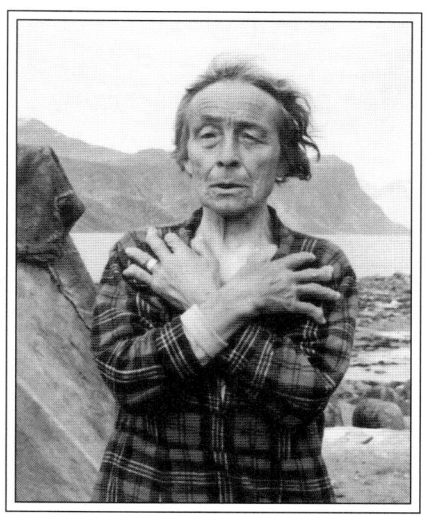

Ashevaq during a visit to Pangnirtung from her home camp of Illongaya in September 1956.

In 1963 Judge John (Jack) Sissons, the first Justice of the Territorial Court of the Northwest Territories, was called to Igloolik island off the Melville Peninsula. He was to decide the fate of three young Inuit charged with helping Kolitalik, the chief of their camp, to commit suicide (Sissons, 1968). Kolitalik, a highly respected and honoured headman, had been in failing health and getting weak. For some reason, he had a terrible fear of losing his mind. He was ready to die and wanted the three young men, one of whom was his son Amah, to help him. Out of respect and loyalty for the beloved patriarch, they agreed to help. They brought in his rifle and Amah loaded it, since his father was too weak to do so. As requested, the three went outside and waited. Then a shot rang out. Kolitalik's wishes had been granted.

In the court case that followed, Judge Sissons declared that all the available evidence indicated that the three men were guilty as charged. But he would not sentence them to punishment of any kind, he said. Justice—including Inuit justice—would be best served by suspending sentence. To do otherwise would be to desecrate the memory of a much-revered headman.

18
Darkness and Light

*Oh, it was wild and weird and wan,
and ever in camp o' nights
We would watch and watch the silver dance
of the mystic Northern Lights.
And soft they danced from the Polar sky
and swept in primrose haze;
And swift they pranced with their silver feet,
and pierced with a blinding blaze.
They danced a cotillion in the sky;
they were rose and silver shod;
It was not good for the eyes of man
—'twas a sight for the eyes of God.*

Robert W. Service (1909:79)

WINTER for the inhabitants of ice-bound Cumberland Sound brought long periods of continuous darkness broken only by a grey, watery twilight that lasted for just a few hours. Even after the sun reappeared in January, the high walls of the fjords kept the whole Pangnirtung settlement in deep shadow during the short daylight hours. The cold was intense. Even though Pangnirtung was 250 km farther south than Aklavik, it felt much colder, something Otto attributed to the high humidity.

But not all was darkness and cold. At times the brilliant northern lights (aurora borealis) shimmered and danced in the sky. Otto even tried to take pictures of the waving bands of yellow, green and silver, but his fingers got numb with the cold. Sometimes great tongues of

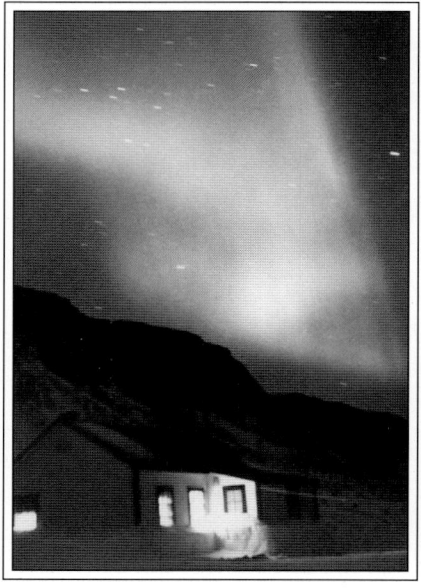 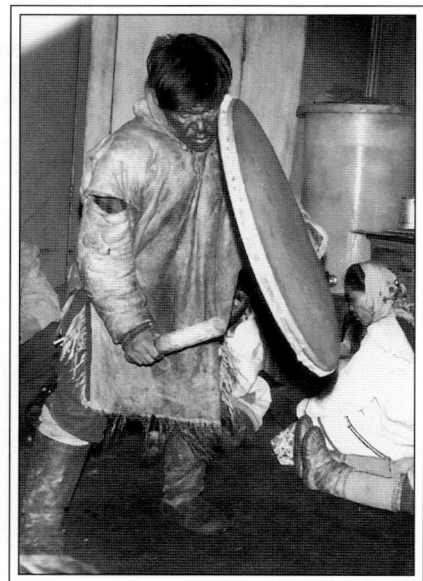

The aurora borealis above the doctor's house in Pangnirtung, February 1956.

A drum dance performed in Arviat (Eskimo Point) by an Ihalmiut from the Kazan River area.

flame seemed to shoot right up to the vault of the sky, only to swirl away and die in an instant. Otto knew the whole grand display was due to "solar particles." But he would never ridicule the Inuit view that the awesome bands and streamers of light were the spirits of their ancestors dancing and playing games on the heavenly plains.

It was also time for dancing on the "earthly plains." When it was too cold or dark to hunt, people gathered to make music. Otto and Didi joined in, surprised to hear an Inuit fiddler playing Scottish tunes and rhythms—a legacy from the Scottish whaling days, they thought. People got up and shuffled along the floor to the tune of "Comin' through the Rye." It may not have been Native folk music, but it produced much gaiety and laughter.

The music was very different from that of the Western Arctic, where the sound—or at least the beat—came from three or four drummers

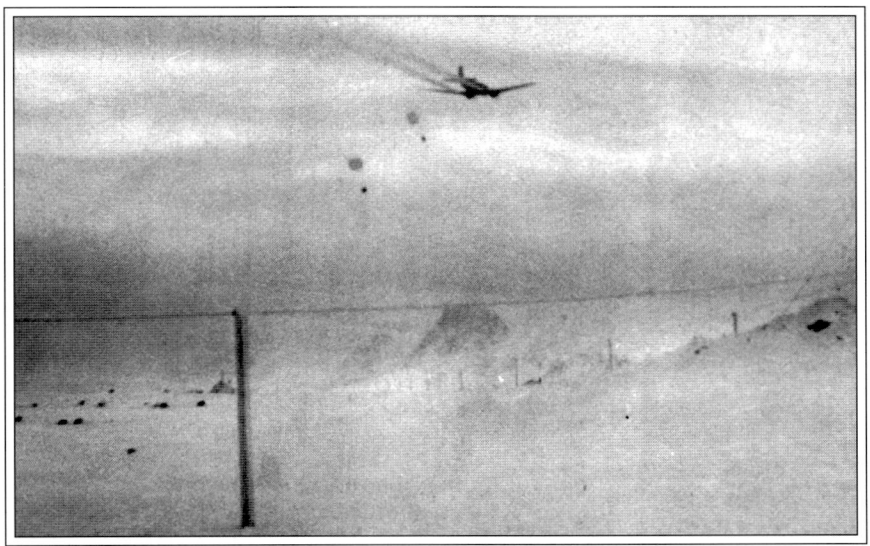

Christmas 1956 parachute drop of mail and Christmas trees by RCAF.

thumping together on drums covered with tightly strung hide. In groups the dancers stomped to the rhythm, swaying from side to side. Sometimes a tune was detectable; sometimes not. And as they drummed away, the men would sing ballads, usually about old legends or successful hunts or fights. They always ended with *Ayaya!*, a word that seemed to convey general approval of it all.

With Christmas, the "gladdest day in all the year," fast approaching, Otto and Didi felt uneasy and wondered what they could tell young Lothar. No trees of any kind could be found on Baffin Island. They could foresee no possibility of having a Christmas tree, an essential part of the German tradition. But the Royal Canadian Air Force came to their rescue on December 19, flying up from Gander, Newfoundland, to drop four Christmas trees by parachute. Bags bulging with Christmas mail and presents were delivered the same way. Otto took pictures of this contemporary "manna from heaven" as it floated down from the sky. Nothing could have brought more excitement to the little community.

94 • Sunrise Over Pangnirtung

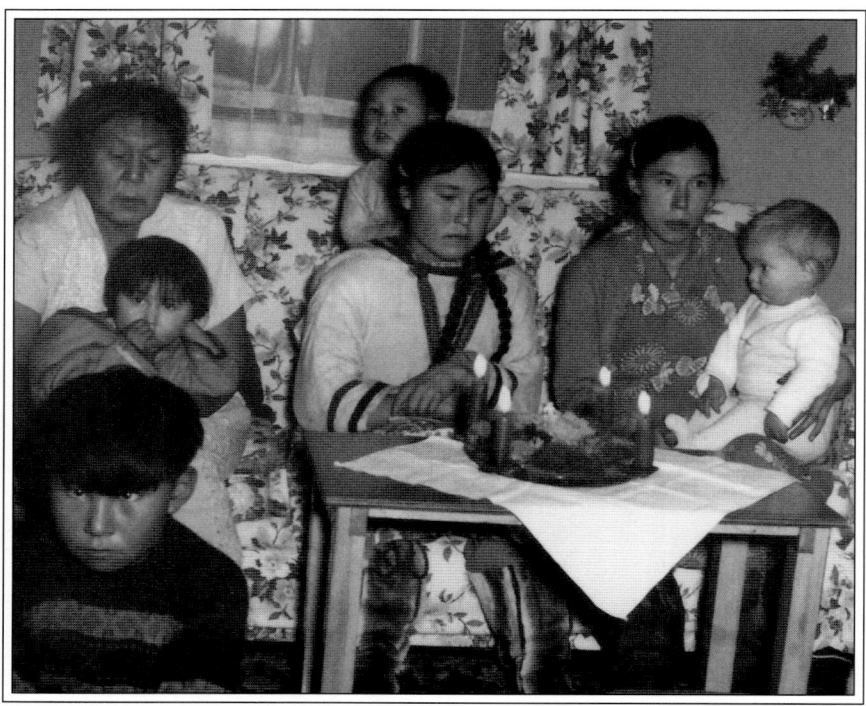

The "Luttamiut" (the doctor's people), visiting the Schaefers' home in Pangnirtung at Christmas. On the left is Etuangat's second wife Nukinga, holding one of her grandchildren. Another grandson sits on the floor in front. Beside Nukinga is the wife of Amosie, the younger son of Etuangat, with her son in her amauti. *On the right is Rosie, the oldest grandchild of Nukinga, holding Alfred, the Schaefers' younger son.*

As Christmas drew near, however, a slight problem arose. Tradition dictated that the doctor's family invite Etuangat and his extended family for Christmas dinner. Otto broached this delicate subject with his wife, knowing the limitations of their little house, and especially of their erratic kitchen stove.

"Can we do it?" he asked with raised eyebrows. (By "we" he meant "you.") "It means feeding at least twenty people, including Rosie and ourselves." Didi nodded her head. Among their supplies delivered by the S.S. *Rupertsland* were a turkey, frozen baked bread, and a few other things. She and Rosie, their Inuit house girl, would cope.

As was the custom in Germany, they decorated the parachuted tree late on Christmas Eve, lit candles, and opened their presents. After the Christmas Day worship service in the Anglican chapel, Etuangat arrived at noon with his wife and the families of his two sons and daughter. Somehow each one of them found a small present under the tree. They dined together, most of the guests sitting on the floor. Everyone thought it was a delicious Christmas dinner; Didi's cookies especially drew a lot of praise.

Etuangat, Amosie, Paulusie, and Taoya and their families were entranced by the Christmas tree decorated with stars and tinsel. They loved the burning candles and the records of German Christmas carols. Otto and Didi were in turn touched by the beautiful presents from their guests. The men brought small ivory carvings—Etuangat's gift was that of a hunter pulling in a harpooned seal. The women gave sealskin mitts and slippers and a small carved bear and seal for Lothar and Alfred. It turned out to be one of the happiest of Christmases, matching the Inuit word for Christmas, *Koviachukbi* (may you be happy).

19
Challenges

LIFE was full, often more than full; both Otto and Didi would have welcomed the proverbial "dull moment." Just feeding themselves and their children, keeping the house warm, hauling in boxes from the storage shed, overseeing the running of the hospital, and giving and receiving radio messages called for the very best they could offer. But the incessant demands on his medical skills challenged Otto more than anything else: they often kept him awake at night, staring at the frost on the ceiling.

Late one night, a baby with seizures was brought in from one of the camps around Cumberland Sound. Norma Westgate, an experienced nurse who had worked with Otto in the All Saints hospital at Aklavik, was on duty and called the doctor. Red-faced and feverish, the sickly infant suddenly jerked into a convulsion and arched its back in spasm. As the anxious father watched, it stopped breathing and turned blue. Then it slowly began breathing again through clenched jaws. Otto gave the baby an injection to control the fits and alcohol sponges to bring down the fever.

Both treatments seemed to be working, but the nurse was not satisfied. "I'll just stay up and watch him," she said. Otto objected. "You can't do that, we've too much to do tomorrow." "All right, but I know what I'll do," said Norma. "I'll lie down with the baby across my chest. If he has another fit, I'll quickly wake up and give him an injection. And I'll be able to tell if he's not breathing properly." And so she passed the night.

The next morning the nurse and her little charge appeared bright and rested. Otto called in the mother, who had stayed overnight in the tent of a villager, and explained that the fits were caused by the baby's high fever. Both doctor and nurse laughed over that night's event, calling it "taking the patient close to your heart!"

Early in 1956, an epidemic of rubella (German measles) swept through parts of Cumberland Sound, including Pangnirtung, killing a number of children. Otto believed it to be the first time that rubella had ever hit Baffin Island. Ordinarily a benign disease (except during pregnancy, when it can cause serious congenital abnormalities in the foetus), here it proved lethal to some children. They lacked the protective antibodies present in groups of people previously exposed to the disease.

Several older people living in camps not far away died from pneumonia and other complications following the epidemic. But what grieved Otto most was the loss of a fit young man, a hunter in the prime of life. Relatives told Otto that the man had had a rash and slight fever before he left to go hunting. But he hadn't seemed very sick and was determined to go out on his own. Sadly, he did not come back. A search party found his body three days later. Otto performed an autopsy and determined that death was due to rampant pneumonia, a sequel to the so-called "mild disease" that was proving so devastating in this virgin population.

But it was the challenges in surgery that taxed Otto as much as anything else. He had acquired some experience in surgery as a junior intern in Edmonton in 1951–52, but certainly not enough to build his confidence. While he was solid in his own specialty, internal medicine, his competence in surgery was "spotty," as he called it. At Aklavik, the experienced Dr. Christensen had done all the operating.

Confident or not, Otto was faced with the need to do an

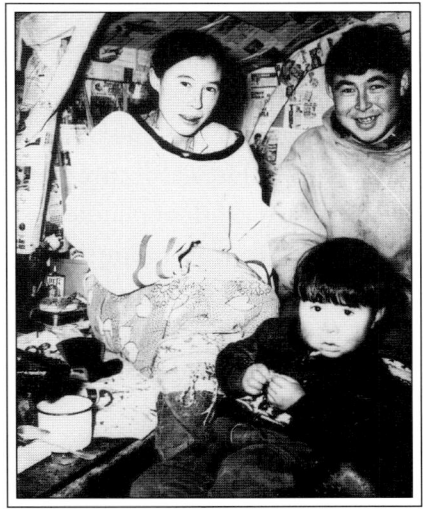

Rosie and her husband Paulusie in their home, which was part tent and part wooden hut. The boy, Guyasie, is the son of Paulusie from his first wife, who died in childbirth.

operation, a Caesarean section, on Rosie, the young woman who worked in the house helping Didi. A tall handsome girl, Rosie was the daughter of an RCMP officer and therefore half-white. She was also the granddaughter of Nukinga, the elderly second wife of Etuangat.

Rosie had been through sad times. After her mother died in childbirth, she was given to the care of various family members. She failed to thrive. Her fortunes improved when she was adopted by Canon John Turner, the celebrated Anglican missionary, and his wife. But the damage had been done: as a little child she had contracted rickets, which left her bones bowed and her pelvis severely deformed. She would never be able to deliver a baby the normal way.

Rosie felt confident as the day for operation drew near, but Otto was awash with apprehension. He called it "a fearsome problem." Before he arrived, the record for two previous Caesarean sections in the hospital was deplorable: in one case, both mother and baby died; in the other, the child was lost. Otto couldn't sleep the night before.

But he had good help. Nurse Vera Roberts would do more than just assist him. Otto had met Vera on board the *C.D. Howe* en route to Pangnirtung. He was impressed, as they prepared for possible surgery on the patient with appendicitis, with how Vera knew her way around the ship's operating room. He also had a good assistant in Didi, who could help with the anaesthesia. But he still felt uneasy, embarking on major surgery in a little hospital that had to rely on melted ice for its water supply and had to sterilize the operating instruments in an ordinary pressure cooker.

The doctor-nurse operating team did the job and did it well. But it might have been otherwise, had Otto not once again demonstrated one of his finest characteristics—a willingness to learn and to be shown. Later he wrote "Vera guided every cut and every step I made," and he was not ashamed to tell others. That day Rosie's eight-and-a-half pound son Billy made his debut, and his mother sailed through the operation. But Otto's foray into major surgery was not yet over. The circulating nurse, Madeleine Salter, uttered those words feared by every surgeon: "A sponge is missing!" Nothing could be more disastrous than leaving a

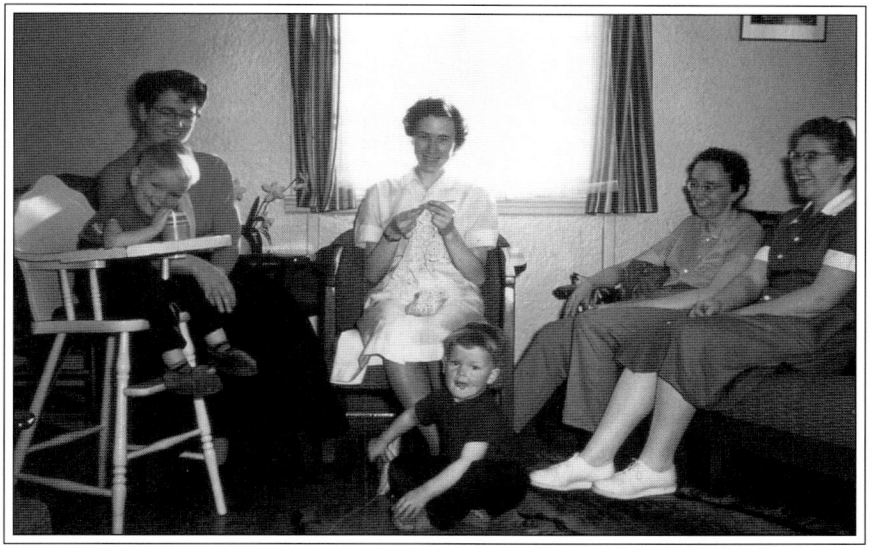

In the sitting room of the Anglican mission house, the home of schoolteacher Dorothy Robinson (second from right). Beside her on the chesterfield is Norma Westgate, head nurse at St. Luke's Hospital. Nurse Vera Roberts is in the middle, and sitting behind Alfred's high chair is Gwen Williams, the hospital cook.

sponge (a sort of towel) inside the patient. They searched and searched and finally had to re-open the incision. The operation took an extra hour, but nothing was found—someone must have made an error in the counting.

Rosie's convalescence was by no means free of worry or concern; she developed a bout of pneumonia and other problems. But she recovered and was soon back in the house helping Didi, while keeping an eye on her healthy, young son. That was all the reward that Otto Schaefer and Vera Roberts needed.

20
Travels by Dog Team

LOOKING back on it all, Otto rates his adventures by dog team over the sea ice or through the rugged hills and valleys of Baffin Island one of the highlights of his life. An emergency call would bring him, Etuangat, and the dogs out any time, except in a blizzard. He tried to plan his non-emergency trips for times when the weather was reasonable, even if unpredictable. With the long winter coming to an end, they would schedule their twice-a-year visits to the 17 camps on the Sound or over the mountains on Davis Strait. Otto estimated that one year the dogs took them on journeys totalling over 2000 km.

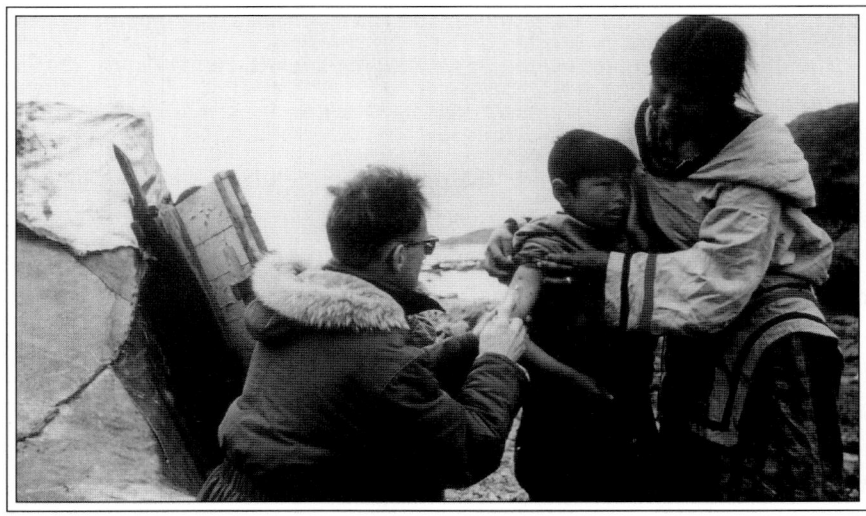

Otto Schaefer giving shots against typhoid fever to camp people in Cumberland Sound, May 1957. Photo taken by Etuangat in camp at Twapait, south of Pangnirtung.

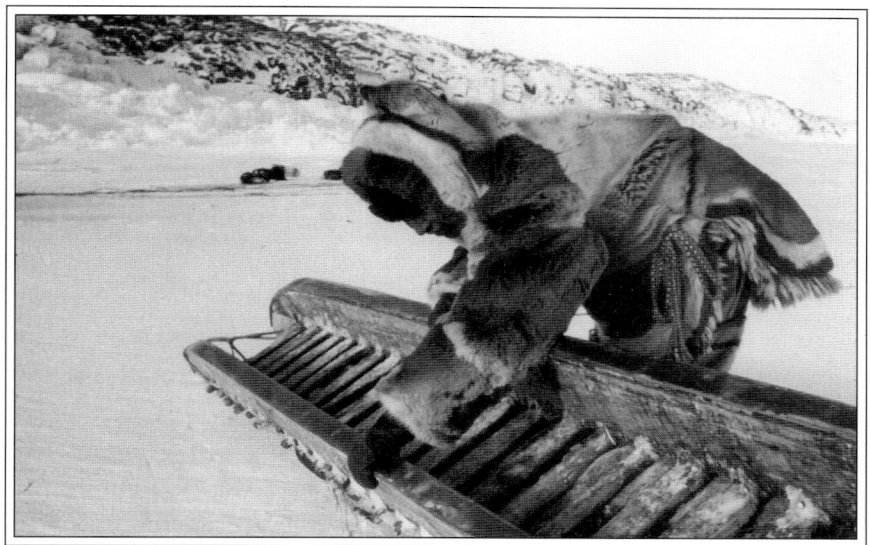

Naudla, from a camp on the northwest coast of Cumberland Sound, overturns his sled to re-ice the steel runners for better gliding at the prevailing temperature of -30°C, February 1956.

Early one morning in March, Otto peeped in at his two sleeping boys, gave Didi a farewell kiss, and set off with Etuangat and his son Amosie on a four-week trip that would take them over the mountains. Amosie's job was to harness the dogs and, after arrival, to feed them, tie them up, and then bed them down in the snow for the night. Leaving on a trip, the strong, thick-chested dogs snarled and nipped at each other in excitement until he buckled them into the security of their harness.

Otto had been tempted to pat or stroke these hard-working dogs, until someone explained that they were not pets. True, Reverend Webster's dogs had saved his life when he got lost in a blinding blizzard. But a savage, hungry dog could be vicious. A few months before, Otto had faced a hideous sight: a five-year-old girl whose face and scalp had been ripped and torn open down to the bone. She was playing with her parents' dog team when the animals attacked her. Otto and the nurses spent four hours resuscitating her and repairing the ugly wounds.

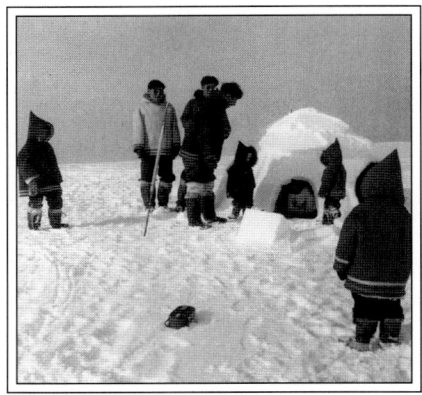

Etuangat (centre) outside the mini-igloo he built for the Schaefer boys and their friends.

On the trail, however, the dogs knew their job and revelled in it. Hauling the heavily loaded *komatik* through the mountain passes to Broughton Island on Davis Strait would require much of their boundless energy, but they seemed to thrive.

The Inuit sled was ideal for the job. According to Etuangat, at one time, whale mandibles had served as runners for the *komatik*. In modern times, the jawbone had been replaced by heavy wooden boards, curved upwards at the front and fitted with metal runners. Early in the winter, the runners were covered with soft mud and put out to freeze. Covered with a thin layer of ice, the frozen mud would allow the sled to glide easily over the hard, windswept, snow of Baffin Island.

On a mild sunny day, travelling by dog team lifted Otto's spirits. But often it was chilly: in spite of his bulky caribou-fur parka and pants and warm *kamiks*, Otto found himself shivering with cold. He would get off the sled and walk briskly beside the dogs, at times running to keep up.

Etuangat was constantly on the move, jumping off his seat on the grub box at the front end. Sometimes it was to dart in among the dogs to free tangled lines, at other times to run in front to steer them away from a jagged ice slab or rock. On a downhill stretch they both hopped off, grabbed a rope dangling from the sled, and dug their heels into the snow. Otto never ceased to be amazed at the stamina and agility of his Inuit friend and helper, almost 20 years his senior. Up well before dawn getting sled and dog team ready, he worked hard all day and remained active and alert. Otto would dearly have liked to borrow some of his boundless energy.

Usually they slept in the tent of a family in the camp they were visiting. On one occasion, they had stopped at the small settlement of Shaunitoratiuk (the place of many bones). There were indeed many bones; most were of sea mammals, but some were human. Otto examined and treated patients until midnight. Then they moved into the large *tupik* (sealskin tent) of Inusilk, the headman, and his family.

The sealskins had been sewn together over a wooden frame. For "windows" two pieces of stretched translucent animal gut allowed some light into the otherwise dark tent. To brighten things up further and add some warmth, Inusilk had tacked up sheets of newspaper and magazines on the sealskin walls. Around the outside of the base of the tent he had packed a foot of thick moss as insulation.

At the back of the *tupik* was the sleeping bench, not much more than a metre and a half wide. The tired visiting team were more than willing to lay their sleeping bags on these thin boards (of priceless value on this treeless island) and collapse inside them.

For Otto it was not a restful night. Every half-hour, their hostess lifted her head to trim the seal-oil lamp, kept burning all night for warmth. The wick, made of arctic cotton grass and willow fibres, needed constant adjusting; sometimes the lamp needed tilting one way or another. Inusilk's wife clearly met one of the chief requirements of a good Inuit wife, described in an Inuktitut proverb: "She must not sleep too soundly; otherwise she will not tend the lamp often enough, and you will freeze or burn with her in your tent." (The other essential was that she should be a good seamstress "or your clothes will rip and tear when you are out hunting.")

On rare occasions that found them out in the wilds with bad weather threatening, Etuangat would build an igloo or snow-house. He had not lost his skill as many others had—in the Eastern Arctic igloos are used on hunting trips, but rarely as a family dwelling. After testing the snow in a drift for depth and firmness, he would cut blocks using his long snow-knife or handsaw, leaving a round, hollow area about three metres wide. Then he piled up the blocks in a spiral ascending towards the dome, trimming them to shape as he went along. Finally, he cut a small opening at snow surface level and built a tunnel for crawling in and out. For ventilation, he jabbed a hollow caribou femur through the top of the igloo. With a seal oil lamp or primus stove burning, an igloo could be amazingly cosy inside, even when a blizzard was raging.

Etuangat always did the cooking. After a couple of days of "white man's food," he would start on what he called "proper food." That often meant cooked seal meat. Even better were the two-inch slabs of frozen raw caribou meat that Etuangat dipped in boiling water just long enough for partial thawing. They often ate raw muktuk, the chewy skin of the beluga whale and the narwhal, a small whale with a peculiar, unicorn-like tusk. Otto grew to enjoy the nutty taste, but wanted to scrape off the layer of unappetizing blubber that was always left on. "You shouldn't be complaining," said Etuangat. "The fat that you think smells so bad is really why the muktuk tastes so good."

Otto's family sometimes had doubts about his frugality and taste for food. He would admonish the children, "You must eat everything. Don't waste a thing." Once he picked a half-rotten tomato from the bottom of the refrigerator and was determined to eat the good half. He had started chewing away on it when the phone rang: one of Otto's old friends was on the line. Five minutes later, Otto hung up, although his friend was still talking away. He had to lie down and looked a bit pale. But he wouldn't admit to anything. "I'm fine. There's nothing wrong with me," he said.

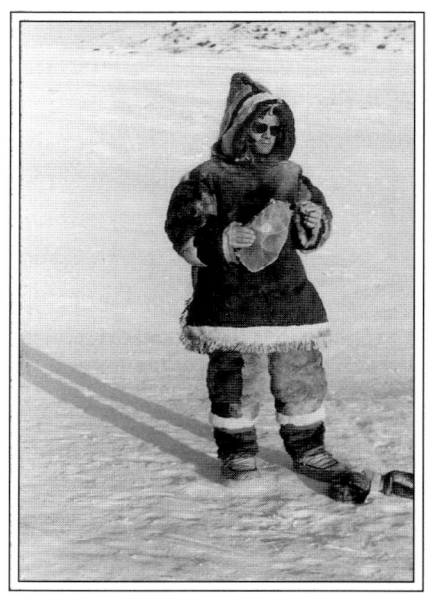

Otto Schaefer eating frozen caribou while travelling by dog team in Kingnait Fiord, south of Pangnirtung in February 1956. Photo by Etuangat.

21
White-Knuckle Moments

It happened one day in April, when Otto was away with the dog team on medical patrol. Etuangat, who usually cut steps in the snowdrifts around the doctor's little house, was also away, and the hard, wind-packed snow piled up. While picking her way carefully over the drifts, Didi, five months pregnant, slipped, fell, and broke her wrist. Worse, she almost immediately felt the ominous cramps of premature labour.

Worried Inuit friends carried her to the hospital. Then the community rapidly mobilized its resources to notify Otto. Using his own and borrowed dogs, the manager of the Hudson's Bay Company trading post assembled a team and harnessed the dogs to a light *komatik*. With two volunteer drivers and six extra replacement dogs running alongside, the rescue mission darted off at top speed. They weren't sure of the route, but knew that the medical patrol had left about eleven hours before for settlements on the west coast of the Sound. Facing a tough assignment, they had one thing in their favour: the day was sunny, clear, and spring-like.

The soft snow of springtime proved to be a blessing in disguise. Otto's dog team and the loaded sled had repeatedly sunk so deep in the snow that the weary dogs had slowed right down. Etuangat figured they were only halfway to Illongaya camp, but it was getting late and they decided to stop for the night. While preparing for their evening meal, they looked up to see "a team with many dogs racing towards us." The panting, exhausted dogs had kept up a torrid pace for five hours. Otto quickly surmised some sort of emergency. A moment later the Inuit driver handed him Vera Roberts' note.

In no time the tired dogs were unhitched and the fresh dogs harnessed up. After a quick cup of tea and biscuits, the two Inuit drivers, with

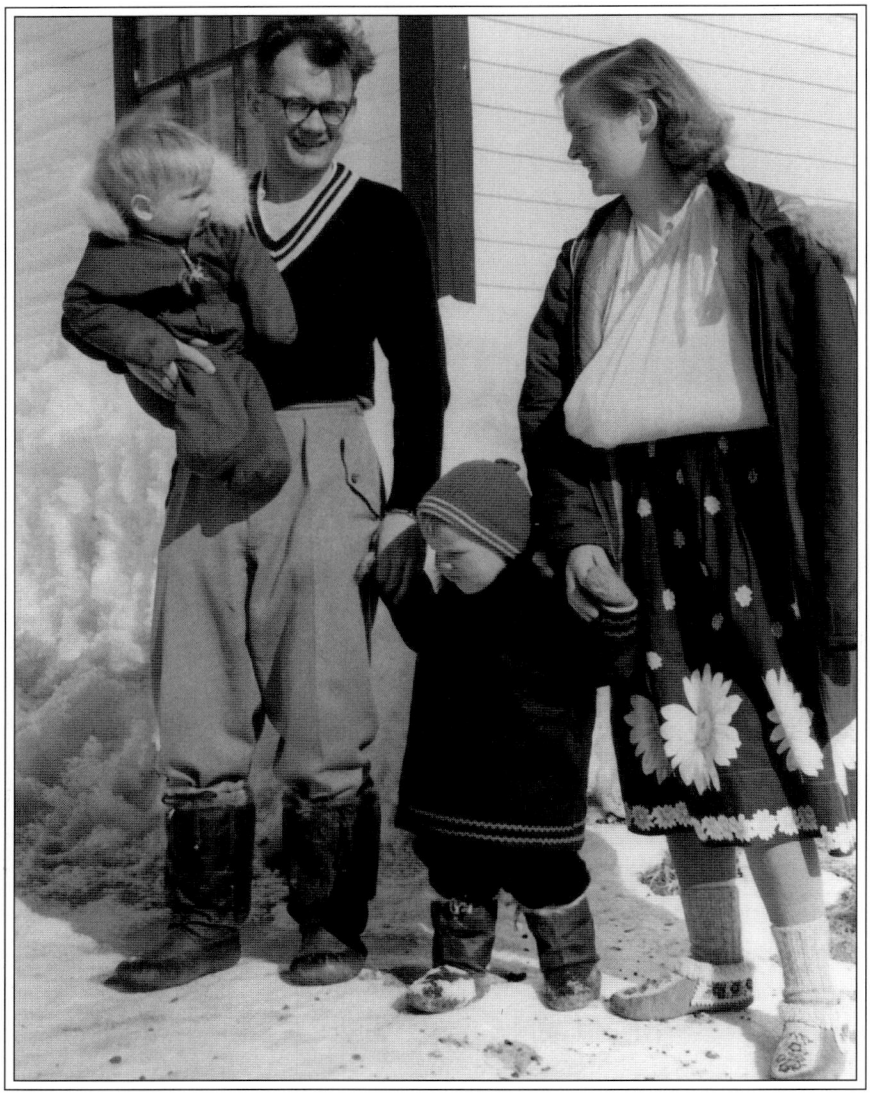

The Schaefer family in April 1956, while Didi was recovering from a fractured wrist.

Otto on board their fast little sled, prepared to hit the trail. A sharp crack of the long whip and couple of "D-r-r-r-r"s spurred the dogs into

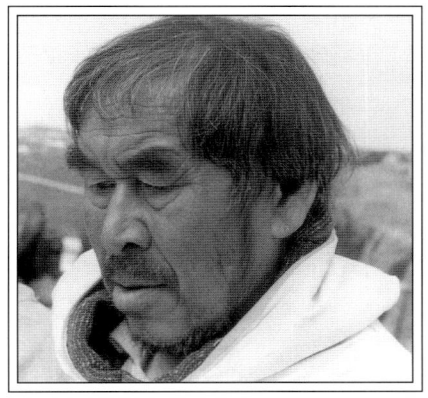

Akshayuk in 1956.

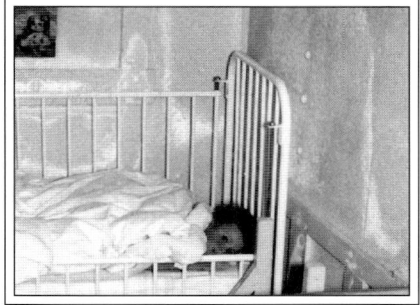

The Schaefer children's room with frost on the walls, February 1956.

action. Sprinting nearly all the way, they made it back to Pangnirtung by 4:00 a.m.

Otto was much relieved to find Didi sleeping soundly in her hospital bed. The premature labour pains had subsided. Once again reliable nurse Vera Roberts had stepped in and done what was required, giving Didi two injections that stopped the contractions. The next day he put her broken wrist in a plaster cast, calling it "a minor problem."

If the comforts and conveniences in the doctor's little cottage left much to be desired, Didi considered the deficiencies were likewise only "minor problems." Family bath night was one of the more unsatisfactory times. Not only was water precious (each person got only three inches), but the collapsible rubber bathtub leaked, and the floor was always cold. Beginning with the boys, each family member went through the procedure of trying to get clean. No one complained, at least not audibly.

One day, however, Didi felt she had plenty to complain about. It was not her usual habit, but early one morning when Otto was away on a dog team patrol, Didi was having a nice leisurely bath in front of the only source of heat, the kitchen stove. Suddenly old Akshayuk, stepfather of Etuangat, barged in carrying coal and barrels of snow and ice. For a few days he was filling in for Etuangat. Stunned at the sight of the intruder, Didi fled soaking wet into the chilly bedroom. Without her towel, she sat there shaking and shivering, while old Akshayuk pottered around for half an hour doing his chores. When she could stand it no longer, she hammered at the door and sent the old man on his way.

Otto heard the story when he returned. He realized that Akshayuk had meant no harm but thought that for Didi's sake, he should ask Etuangat to talk to the old man. The outcome surprised Otto. Akshayuk simply could not under-stand why the naked Didi should have run away into the bedroom. After all, he was just a harmless old man. Besides, the Inuit think there is nothing wrong with seeing a female breast: they look upon it as an organ for feeding babies, not a sexual organ. Otto agreed. Didi was not so sure, but they both had a good laugh. Later Otto expressed the wish that our Western society might adopt the Inuit's sensible attitude towards the female bosom.

On August 11, 1956 a beautiful, fair-haired daughter was born to Didi and Otto, a sister for Lothar and Alfred. They had already chosen a name for her; in fact, there was never any doubt. She would be given the same name as Etuangat's daughter: Taoya (pronounced "Towya"). According to Inuit custom, a child is not given the name of a friend or relative without permission. Although Etuangat "didn't believe in that old non-sense," he did suggest asking his daughter. The adult Taoya, a young mother in her twenties, said she would be honoured. In the Inuktitut language, Taoya means "clear of vision." The name would later seem remarkably appropriate.

Baby Taoya thrived in the Arctic. In spite of the chilly environment of their little house, the children kept warm at night with woolen socks and warm comforters. Didi made mitts for baby Taoya and tied them on with laces. But one night Taoya extracted one hand from her mitt and froze her little finger. The deformity is still there to remind her of Pangnirtung, her birthplace.

22
Allies, Most of the Time

In their efforts to relieve suffering and hardships and upgrade the quality of life of the Inuit, the health care team worked with three allies: the Hudson's Bay Company trading post, the RCMP, and the Mission. Otto Schaefer enjoyed good relations and cooperation with all three—most of the time. For example, Shorty Tinling, the manager of the Hudson's Bay Company post, was at the forefront of the community's efforts to send a rescue team to find Otto after Didi's accident.

Without the Anglican Mission hospital at Pangnirtung, Otto would have been handcuffed in his work to care for the sick and injured. He

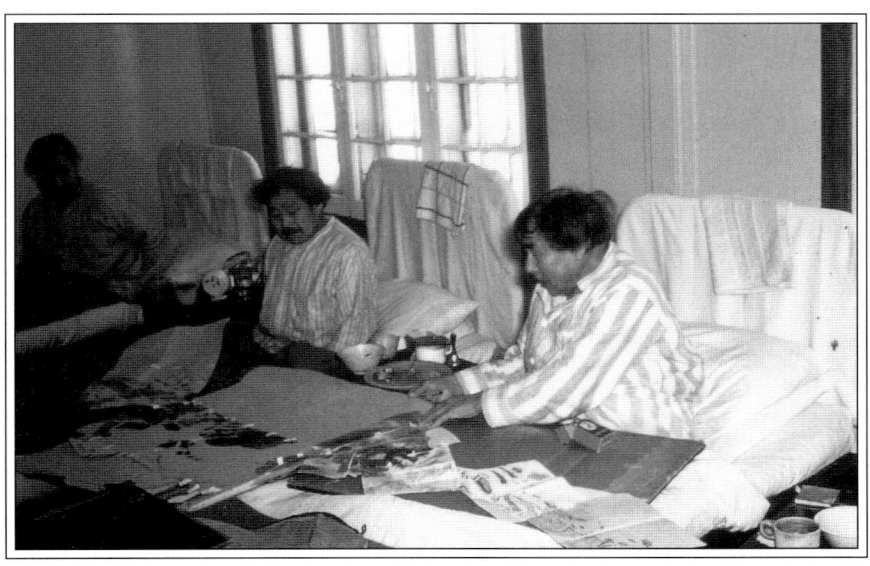

The men's tuberculosis ward in St. Luke's Hospital, Pangnirtung, February 1956.

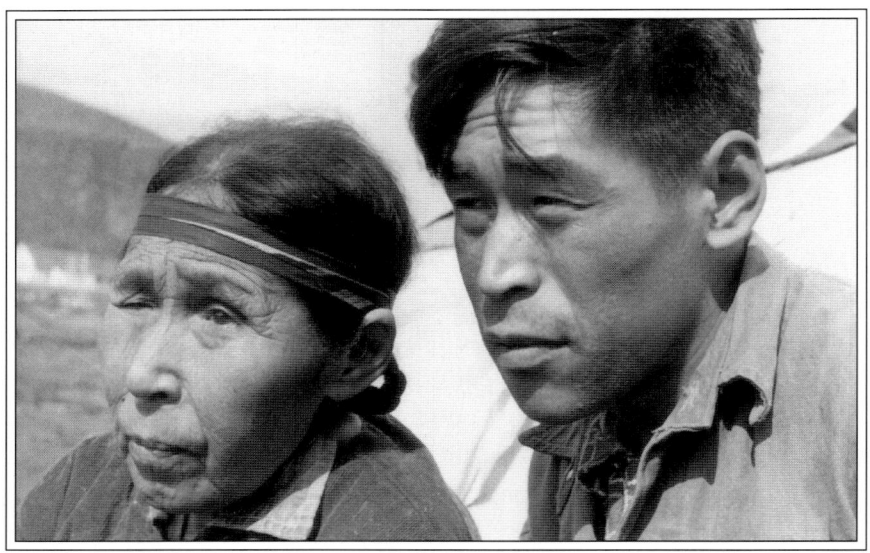

Joanasie (right) with Utaluk, his mother-in-law, in 1956. Joanasie helped out at the hospital.

went on record as saying: "This little hospital does excellent work." He admired Norma Westgate and Vera Roberts, devoted and industrious nurses who worked all day and then cared for emergencies at night. He liked the way they moved so freely and easily with the Inuit people. He found he could rely on the Inuit nurse-aides, who got their training on the job.

All the people of Pangnirtung claimed to be Christian, although some, like Etuangat, retained their belief in the *angakok* or medicine man. In fact, the entire Native population of Baffin Island had become Christian, and most people took seriously their new-found Anglican faith.

Otto found out that the inhabitants of Hoare Bay at the east end of Cumberland Peninsula venerated the Sabbath. Arriving there on a Saturday night, he had hoped to examine patients on Sunday afternoon after the morning worship service. But the headman shook his head, saying that the community devoted the whole day to worship, singing, and praying.

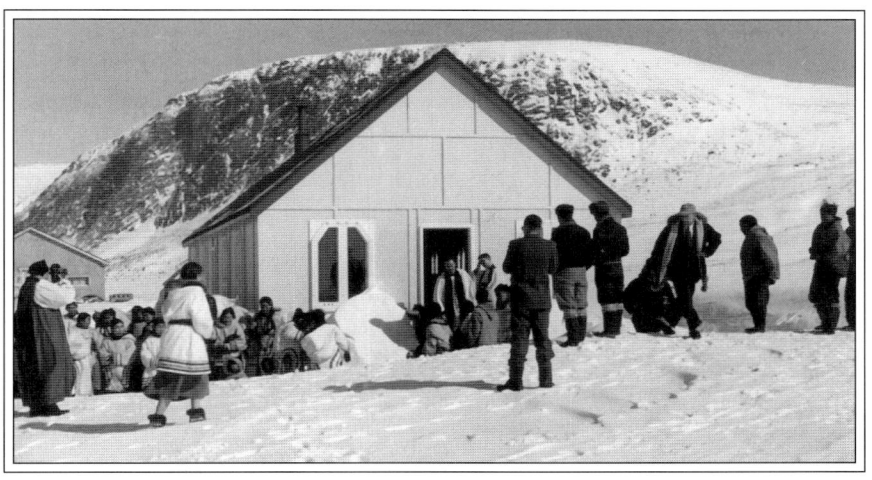

Bishop Donald Marsh (left) taking pictures after the inauguration of the new Anglican Church in Pangnirtung on April 21, 1957.

Otto took exception to an article about missionaries in Inuit life published in the *Canadian Magazine* a few years later. In a written reply, he objected strongly to the statement: "The white man has introduced the Inuit to problems of ethics and morality that could make him neurotic" (Hicks, 1972). Otto went on to say that the missionaries "did much to protect Eskimos against some of the worst abuses and exploitation by whalers, trappers, and traders; filled a real void when the old animistic ghost world collapsed; and prepared Eskimos as best they could for onslaught of military (DEW line), government, and industrial [oil-mineral] development which, wanted or not, came their way" (Schaefer, unpubl. letter).

Otto and Didi particularly enjoyed the friendship of the Reverend and Mrs. Smythe, Anglican missionaries who had come out of retirement to fill in at Pangnirtung for three years. Elderly but vigorous and active, Mr. Smythe also took on the job of building a much-needed extension to the hospital and nurses' quarters. Mrs. Smythe, whom Otto described as "an excellent cook," often invited the doctor and his family to her home for meals.

Like most people on Baffin Island, Otto and Didi had heard the tragic story of the legendary Anglican priest, Canon John Turner. In 1929 he had begun ministering to the Inuit of Baffin Island, learning their language and teaching literacy. The people loved and revered him for his sincerity and practical caring. A muscular man as rugged as the land, he travelled long distances by dog team to visit Inuit settlements, shooting game to feed himself and his dogs. In 1944 he returned to England to marry a nurse and brought her back to remote and isolated Moffet Inlet, not far from Arctic Bay at the north end of Baffin Island.

On September 30, 1947, Turner's name flashed over the airwaves across Canada. A week before he had been out seal hunting. Back at home, the trigger of his .22 rifle snagged in his clothes and fired a bullet through his face and into his brain. Paralyzed and in pain, he remained mentally alert and just able to speak. News of the accident reached Army headquarters in Ottawa. In a most heroic and dangerous rescue mission that overcame seemingly insurmountable obstacles, the Canadian Army and Air Force succeeded in rescuing Turner. But the mortally injured man did not get to a hospital in Winnipeg until 52 days after the accident. John Turner died two weeks later from meningitis, a complication of his brain injury. A previously unsung hero, he left a legacy of goodwill amongst his Inuit friends. Twenty-five years later, his courageous wife went back to Baffin Island for five years; two of her daughters also returned to the North to teach and to nurse (Halliday, 1995).

Otto Schaefer had been on good—even friendly—terms with the local RCMP officer, until one day a scowling Corporal Barr approached him with a summons in his hand. Some weeks previously, Otto and Etuangat had come across a large collection of human skulls and other bones near Kingnait Fiord, just east of Pangnirtung. Because permafrost makes burial impossible, bodies are usually placed in boulder cairns. Etuangat thought a large settlement had once existed at the site but had been abandoned long ago. (It was an old Thule site, which had been mentioned by Boas.)

Otto found a mummified human leg there. He removed a tiny fragment and sent it to Ottawa for carbon dating. The human tissue was estimated to be at least 500 years old. Interested in physical anthropology for several years, he picked up one skull that intrigued him. For one thing, the bony ridge down the middle of the inside was unique. For another, the jaw had no teeth and the sockets were worn down, suggesting the person had lost his or her teeth during life. This finding, which pointed towards dental caries, contradicted current belief that there was no tooth decay among the Inuit until candy and pop came along.

Etuangat gave his opinion that there was nothing culturally offensive in Otto's sending the skull for examination to Dr. R.S. MacNeish, anthropologist at the National Museum in Ottawa. Dr. MacNeish had previously given Otto a set of calipers and shown him how to measure skulls. Otto boxed up the skull for shipment. Then he sent a telegram, saying the skull was to be a gift to the Museum.

Unfortunately for Otto, the contents of the telegram fell into the law-enforcing hands of Corporal Barr, who appeared in uniform early one morning to charge Otto with desecration of a human burial site. Barr confiscated the skull and ordered Otto to appear in court before the local Justice of the Peace. But the Justice of the Peace was Otto, who was also Coroner. If he was absent (or in this case, the accused), then the local schoolteacher, Dorothy "Robbie" Robinson, was to take over. After hearing the evidence, Robbie pondered for a few minutes, and then dismissed the case.

The RCMP wouldn't give up that quickly, however. This was a serious matter, and they appealed. Otto was beginning to wonder about the seriousness of his crime. He contacted his Edmonton lawyer, Mr. Gerald Amerongen, whose family had been so kind to the new immigrants from Germany back in 1951. Mr. Amerongen suggested Otto find out the exact nature of the offence he had committed. After some time, when Mr. Amerongen contacted Inspector Larson, head of the RCMP, he was told that the case had been dropped.

Paradoxically, instead of having to wear the ignoble mantle of desecrator of human remains, Otto went on to become a "preserver." At his request, the appropriate department in Ottawa declared the prehistoric site in Kingnait Fiord, with its large collection of burials, to be a designated historical site. Otto proved to be respectful of bones after all.

23
Hunting and Survival

For the inhabitants of the frozen North, no activity was more important than hunting and no one was more respected than a good hunter. Hunger and famine always lurked nearby. Most of the older people could tell stories—often human tragedies—of times when they had faced starvation.

When the caribou herds suddenly changed their migration routes and disappeared from areas of the Central Arctic in the 1940s, famine hit parts of the Keewatin District, especially the Arviat (Eskimo Point)

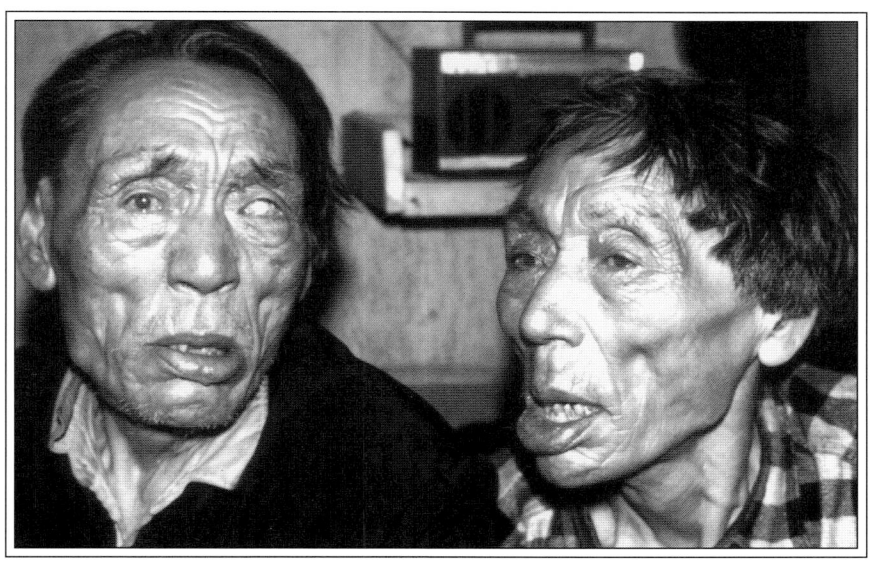

Two survivors of Padlermiut Inuit who survived the famine in the south Keewatin District in the 1940s. Over 100 lives were lost when the caribou migration routes changed.

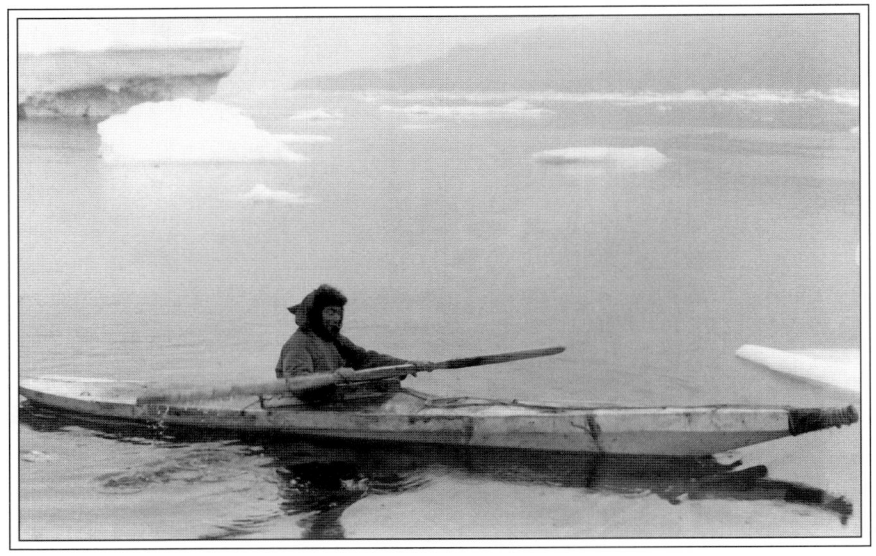

A kayaker in Cumberland Sound, July 1956.

area. Many children and old people died. Otto had heard much about the disaster that had befallen people near Cape Dyer at the south end of Baffin Island. His patient, Tapitia, was the sole survivor. An entire settlement had been snuffed out after a monstrous fall of heavy snow that put a stop to any hunting.

Fishing and hunting sea mammals provided the basic food resources for Inuit in coastal areas, and one day Otto found out what it was like to hunt for whales. Whaling had once been a major industry in the Eastern Arctic, dominated by Scottish and American whalers. They had almost wiped out the whale population in the area by the time the International Whaling Commission imposed a ban in 1946. In the Cumberland Sound area, the Inuit still hunted the *killaluga* (beluga or white whale), an animal five metres long that weighed up to 900 kg.

"It was different in the old days," said Etuangat, as they cruised along in a powerboat to an area where beluga schools had been spotted. "When whales were heading up the fiord, we followed behind them in *kayaks* and *umiaks*, shouting and hollering. When they got up to shallow water, we would beat the water with paddles and keep them there until the tide went out. Then we could get close enough to harpoon them." But it could be risky and sometimes, as Etuangat casually mentioned, the whale won the battle.

In a relatively fast motorboat and armed with rifles it should be easy, Otto thought. But it proved to be a tricky business. In the strong wind, white-capped waves tended to hide the whales. Fortunately by midnight the sea had calmed, and the boats started to circle around the beluga schools. Then the hunters fired a salvo of shots, not at the whales but into the air. "You'll see why," said Etuangat.

The whales dived and disappeared for what seemed a long time. When they resurfaced to take a long gulp of air, they exposed themselves to the hunters, ready with rifles cocked. They fired to wound, not to kill: it seemed inhumane, but a fatally shot whale would sink and be lost. Wounding the animal with several body shots would weaken it so that it would have to come up for air more often. Otto watched as the boats closed in and the hunters harpooned the wounded whales. The harpoon was connected to an air-inflated sealskin buoy that prevented the animal from diving deep again.

The Inuit considered the rifle a tool to provide their essential food, not a weapon to attack others. On that day, Etuangat, his son Amosie, and his son-in-law Paulusie shot and killed three whales and towed them back to a small sheltered bay, where they started to skin them at about 2:00 a.m.

Suddenly a blustery squall interrupted their work, and they decided to head for home. They didn't get far before powerful wind gusts and churning waves threatened to hurl them against the rocks. They gave up and sought shelter in the little cove of Awataktuk, west of Pangnirtung. For two full days they sheltered there before returning home with their quarry. Didi was glad and relieved to see the hunters back safe and fairly sound—the same violent storm had struck Pangnirtung. She had feared the low-risk expedition was turning into a nightmare.

The whales were butchered, and almost all parts were used. For the next few days, many hands worked at scraping the blubber from the

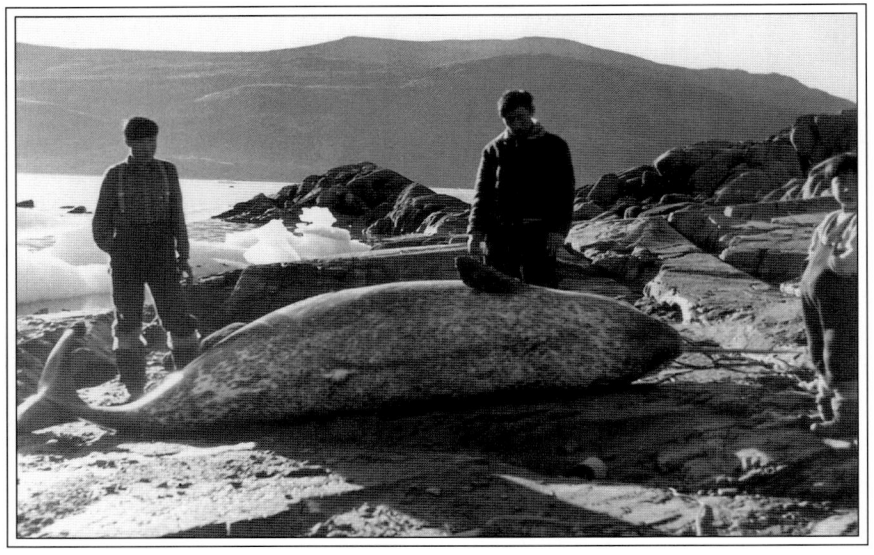

Etuangat (right) with his son Amosie, behind a narwhal shot at the entrance to Pangnirtung Fiord in August 1957.

whale skins. Otto had to treat some of these hands that got nicked and cut. Chunks of blubber were thrown into barrels for rendering into oil and eventual shipment to Montreal for margarine production. Slabs of skin were sent to England to make shoelaces.

Seals were actually a far more important source of food and clothing than whales, even if hunting them was less of an adventure. In spring, hunters needed only to go down to the edge of the ice floe where the tides had created openings in the ice. Scraping the ice was usually enough to bring up the seal, a curious animal. But as with whales, the hunter had to be quick to harpoon the wounded seal or it would sink. When the Sound was frozen over, a hunter had to wait patiently by a seal's breathing hole. When the seal came up for air, the hunter could use a spear or rifle.

Not an ounce of the seal was wasted: the hide was used to make tents and *kamiks* (boots), the blubber was rendered into oil for lamps, and the meat was eaten. The intestine—carefully washed out, of course—

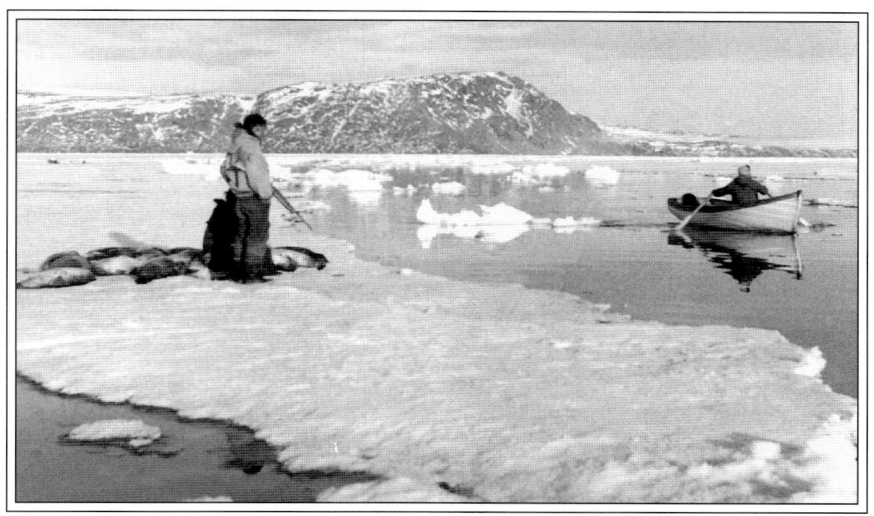

Etuangat's son Amosie standing beside a pile of shot seals in late June 1956.

was considered a delicacy. In keeping with his eclectic tastes, Otto thoroughly enjoyed it.

Everyone wore sealskin boots, but there was one problem: they had to be chewed. After frequent soakings in snow and water, they tended to get hard and uncomfortable to wear. The task of chewing the boots of their husbands and sons to keep them soft and pliable fell to the women. A good Inuit mother and wife might spend hours at this job, and the constant chewing eventually wore her teeth down to stumps. It was hard work, but she was well rewarded by the thanks of her family. Furthermore, although her teeth wore down, they did not decay.

If they wanted walrus, hunters had to travel by boat to a group of distant islands. The meat had two disadvantages: it contained 10 percent fat, and it sometimes gave rise to trichinosis, a disease caused by a parasite. But it was excellent for dog food, providing the extra energy the dogs needed. Polar bear meat was even more dangerous: almost half of the great white animals were infested with trichinosis. After 20 people died in the Cape Dorset area of Baffin Island one year, investigations revealed they had eaten partially cooked polar bear meat.

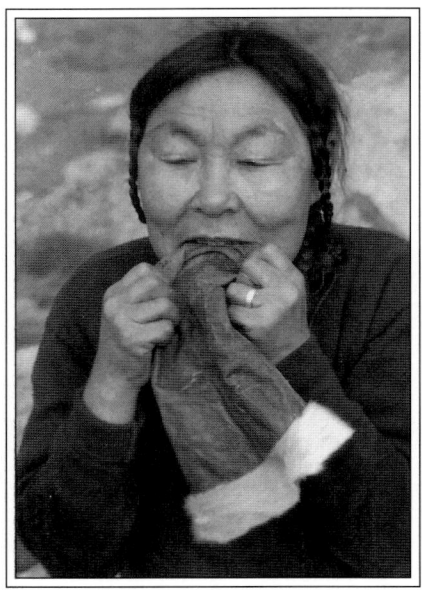

Samonie chewing on a kamik *(sealskin boot) to soften it.*

Although the Inuit had to kill animals to keep themselves alive, a curious sort of bond and warm feeling existed between the people and their game. Etuangat described an old custom: taking a bite from the warm liver of a freshly killed animal. The hunter considered the liver to be the seat of the creature's soul and spirit. By eating it, he showed respect for and reconciliation with his victim.

Known among Indians and Europeans as "eaters of raw meat," the Inuit rarely suffered from malnutrition. In the summer and fall, they collected small quantities of berries and roots. Seaweed scraped from the rocks in the high tidal areas provided a source of vitamins far richer than most vegetables. Even the partly digested contents of stomach and upper intestine of butchered caribou and arctic hare were eaten, in spite of bitter stomach acid. By eating much of their meat or fish raw or half-cooked, they avoided vitamin deficiencies.

Otto and Didi's children thrived on Inuit food. Lothar was never happier than when gnawing on a chunk of seal meat. Baby Alfred, when not quite two, found other delicacies. One day his mother, cleaning an Arctic char, had severed the fish's head, which fell to the floor. Before Didi knew it, Alfred had crawled along the floor, poked out the eyes, and eaten them. He was only doing the same as his friends living in nearby sealskin tents—they competed for the eyes and brain as the choicest bits.

Fresh oranges came by boat only once a year. Otto thought there must be a good way to preserve them for the winter. It was easy enough

Hunting and Survival • 121

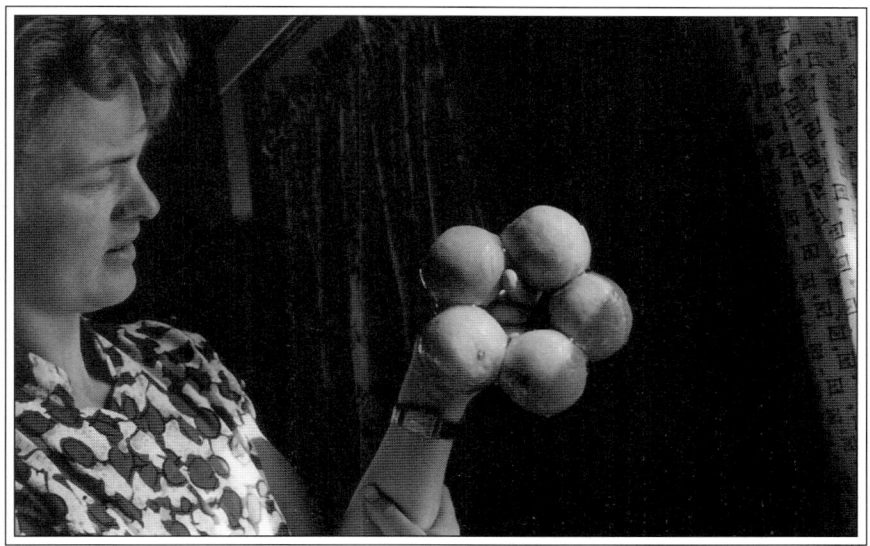

Didi Schaefer with oranges that had been frozen all winter.

to freeze them and keep them frozen, but what would they be like when thawed? Didi learned that if they were thawed slowly in a pot of cold water, they kept their form and shape (and more importantly, their taste). She felt she had made a major discovery: a source of fresh fruit during the long months of canned food.

If food—and not money—dominated the thoughts and actions of the hardy Baffin Island people, they would not bend the rules to get it. During the winter of 1956–57, the thermometer outside the Schaefer house plummeted to -52°C. The salt water of the entire length of Cumberland Sound froze solid, a rarity that had not occurred for over fifty years. As a result, seal hunting was almost impossible, ice fishing on inland lakes uncertain, and caribou hunting likewise precarious. People living in settlements at the west end of the Sound faced dwindling food stocks.

Some desperate hunters came down to the Pangnirtung area, hoping for better luck. Well aware of their plight, Otto asked Etuangat to tell them to go into the warehouse for the doctor and his family. There was plenty of food there; they could help themselves. Etuangat did so, but two weeks passed and not one item of the food stocks had been taken. Otto wondered what to do next and asked Etuangat for his advice.

"You need to go along with them to the warehouse and hand things out to them personally," he said. "They'll never take anything on their own, no matter how hungry they are."

Their complete trustworthiness deeply impressed Otto. But so did other qualities, such as their willingness to share. "The unlucky hunter will not starve as long as a luckier neighbour can be reached," he once wrote. He had found out—by suffering Etuangat's rebuke—how children learn from infancy by imitating their parents and working together without coercion. He had also observed the complete interdependence within the extended family, along with extreme personal tolerance. On many a day, Otto found himself contrasting the society of his Inuit friends with Western society, where individual interests dominate and displace family priorities, to the detriment of all. It's no wonder he declined the invitation to leave Pangnirtung to join his friend's medical practice in British Columbia.

24
"The Arctic We Knew"

Early in June 1957, winter launched its final fling at Cumberland Sound, dumping almost 40 centimetres of snow on Pangnirtung in one night. Then a brisk rainfall seemed to devour all the snow, leaving deep pools of water everywhere. Covered with fresh meltwater, the sea ice appeared to be thawing, but it would take much more warm sun to melt ice almost two metres thick.

Spring had come. One of the surest sounds of spring was the wild roaring of the river, still hidden under snow and ice. The tumbling water bored an ever-larger channel as it flowed from the rolling plateau

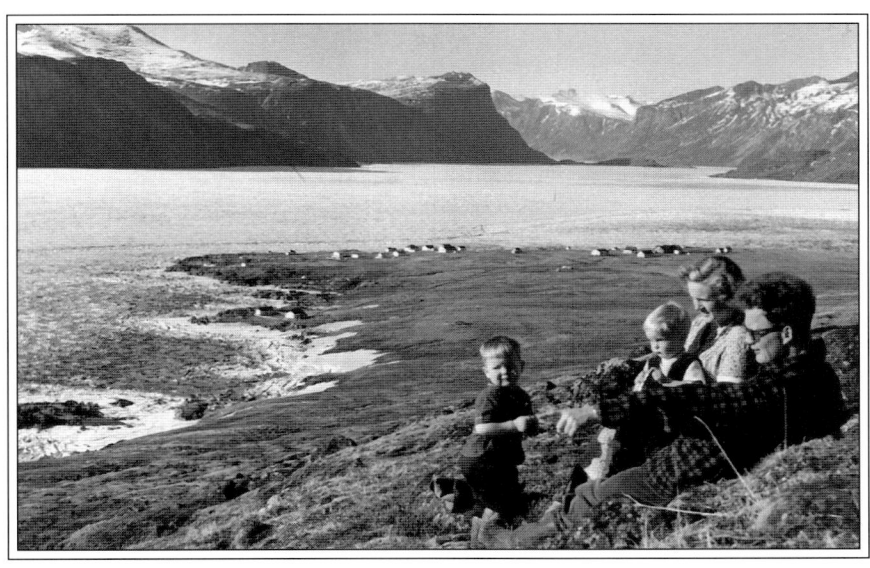

The Schaefers having a picnic on the slopes above Pangnirtung in late June 1956.

above the fjord down to the sea. In a few days, it would break out of its winter shell. Then foaming white torrents would cascade down, spraying fine droplets that broke up the rays of the round-the-clock sunshine into rainbows. Overhead, squadrons of white snow geese winged their way north to their summer nesting areas. The time of day didn't matter—you could go berry-picking at 3:00 a.m. if you wanted to. Otto and Etuangat did just that, gathering juicy blueberries and crowberries that the snow had nicely preserved all winter. But the berries had to be picked as they emerged from the melting snow; otherwise, the birds or the sun would finish them.

Otto wondered which of the two locations was the most inimical for growing plants or trees: the Sahara Desert or Baffin Island. Not until the end of July would tundra flowers finally bloom, far later than in Aklavik.

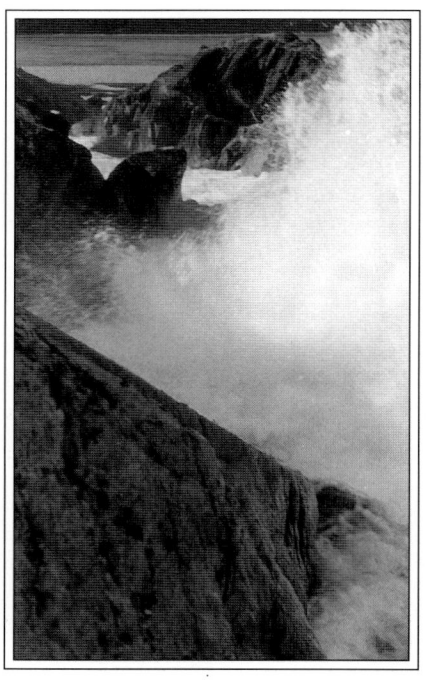

A waterfall on the river, about 1 km above Pangnirtung.

Otto had encountered several fragile shoots of arctic willow (*Salix arctica*) about five centimetres high and found that they were connected to a central stem the thickness of his thumb. He cut across the stem with an axe and tried to count the number of rings with a magnifying glass, but they were too tiny. Later he learned that the little arctic willows may grow up to shoulder height under favourable conditions. Botanists have determined that some of these small shrubs are several hundred years old.

Didi and Otto had looked forward to hiking and picnic outings during their last months at Pangnirtung, but it was not to be. On a sunny afternoon in May,

Didi fell while skiing on the slope above the settlement and broke her leg, sustaining a spiral fracture of the tibia. Otto did his best to correct the displacement and put her leg in a plaster cast, knowing that she really needed to be evacuated to Montreal for orthopaedic care. Norma Westgate helped Otto to make the decision: "You'll be blaming yourself for the rest of your life if she is left with a limp." It was as hard to get Didi out of Pangnirtung as it was to get her back home again. She was away from May until August.

Then it was time to think of leaving. How they would have loved to stay on. True, the contract had been for a two-year period, but they wondered: couldn't it be prolonged? Didi, who had missed the summer activities of both those years (she was in the latter stage of pregnancy during their first summer), insisted that Otto ask for an extension. Otto complied, only to learn that his successor, Dr. Sabine, was already on board the *C.D. Howe* and would reach Pangnirtung in a few weeks. Disappointed, they resigned themselves to moving on.

One day in September, Otto and Didi paddled a canoe down Pangnirtung Fiord to the area where it joined the Sound. Already winter seemed to be hovering nearby. Chill winds from the south had blown in thick ice floes that had drifted down from the High Arctic with the Labrador Stream. Paddling in and around the great masses of floating ice, the Schaefers too felt a part of the scene. It wasn't beautiful, or warm, or comforting—but it was magnificent.

Otto came close to dropping warm tears on the page of his diary when he wrote at the time of departure: "Our boys were sad when they learned their friends could not come along. Didi and I tried to hide our sadness." It was hard to say *Tabawutit* (good-bye) to Etuangat, Nukinga, Rosie, Amosie and their families.

The night before they boarded the ship, the evening concert of howling dogs lulled them to sleep for the last time. During the early days at Pangnirtung, Otto had found himself annoyed by the melancholy baying and howling of one group of dogs and the long, wailing reply from another. But later he felt a curious sense of peace. The image of such a dog, head turned high and howling its woes into a flaming red

Arctic sunset, would always speak to the Schaefers of "our own longing for the Arctic we knew and loved."

25
Turning Point

OCTOBER 1957 found Otto back in Edmonton at the Charles Camsell Hospital for Indians and Inuit. At first he worked as a general physician, but later he was given responsibility for patients on the Internal Medicine wards. He was in a sense retracing old steps, but he chose to make it a time for consolidation and moving forward. After the experience of Aklavik and Pangnirtung, he was ready to move on. During the ensuing months he worked with respected consultants like Dr. Allan M. ("Buzz") Edwards. Later Dr. Edwards would describe his junior colleague as "a warm individual with a great capacity for friendship; Native people revered him, recognizing in him genuine interest and sincerity."

Nurse Kay Dier remembers some of Otto's "interesting theories," one of which she considered just a bit weird. Otto speculated that Inuit living near Spence Bay got more cancer because of their proximity to the magnetic pole. "He seemed to bubble over with new and imaginative ideas," she said.

Nurse Emmi Nemetz remembers that Otto corrected a common misconception that Inuit can tolerate pain that would be agony for others. "Just because they are quiet and not shouting for a needle does not mean they are not suffering," he said. He too had once misinterpreted silence as indicating a high pain threshold. "After Otto came back from the North," said Emmi, "patients got the drugs for pain after surgery without having to ask or wait."

Feeling the need to be recognized in his specialty in Canada, Otto applied for study leave the following July and spent a year at the University Hospital across the river. The Canadian Royal College had given him little recognition for the years of specialty training in Germany. Thanks to Dr. Edwards, he was given credit for one of the years he had spent working at the Camsell. Looking back, he feels grateful for the time on the wards at the University Hospital as an assistant resident with superb consultants like Dr. Allan Gilbert and Dr. Dick Rossall. In 1963 he wrote and passed the certification exam in internal medicine, and he was awarded the Fellowship diploma a year later.

In January 1958, Otto and Didi had stood before a magistrate in Edmonton and pledged their allegiance to the country that had been their home for seven years. They felt happy to be New Canadians, as they were called, but later that year something happened to make Otto wish he were not a German-Canadian. His friend Dr. Helmut Reubsatt had repeatedly invited Otto to move to Castlegar, British Columbia to join him in a busy family practice. Both Otto and Didi loved the Arctic and planned to go back north, but it was hard to ignore Dr. Reubsatt's invitation. When he wrote about "our big lake near the mountains," they just had to go and see for themselves.

On the way to Vancouver during a fall holiday, they travelled to Castlegar. They found it to be a beautiful place, but they were still ambivalent. Otto decided to visit the Vancouver office of the B.C. College of Physicians and Surgeons. He would have to register with the College if they moved to Castlegar.

Otto appeared before the committee of the College that interviewed new doctors. The registrar reviewed his credentials and references and supported his application. But other members of the committee spoke strongly against him. It felt like a punch to the stomach to be told, "You've got a horrible German accent, and we don't need doctors like you in B.C." That unhappy episode closed the Castlegar door once and for all, and in a way Otto and Didi felt relieved. But it also reminded them that memories of World War II were still smouldering 13 years later.

Part of Otto's nature as a child was a consuming curiosity, a burning desire to know, to study, and to look beyond the apparent for underlying causes and reasons. Otto's mother had said, "The other children ask what is this and what is that, and I give them an answer. But you always want to know why."

In Aklavik, Otto was constantly writing in a little notebook. At the ports of call visited by the *C.D. Howe*, he examined hundreds of patients, entering in a large record book their state of health, diet and nutrition, history of family illnesses, and lifestyle. He compared the health of Inuit living, for example, at Cape Dorset on Baffin Island with those on Ellesmere Island farther north. At each port he seized every opportunity to talk to young and old, Mounties, priests, traders, and trappers. He documented all the information he considered to be of value.

He published his first paper (in English) in the August and September 1959 issues of the *Canadian Medical Association Journal* (CMAJ), under the title "Medical Observations and Problems in the Canadian Arctic, Parts I and II" (Schaefer, 1959). This 14-page article became a classic against which other publications on this subject would be measured. For Otto, it was the first of over 100 contributions to the medical literature.

He began the article by giving his reasons for writing: the need to better understand health problems as the North increased in importance, the lack of any previous systematic studies of the health of the Inuit by doctors working year-round in the Arctic, and the impact on the primitive northern society of burgeoning "civilization."

He referred to his travels by dog team, the battle against tuberculosis, the terrible epidemics of measles, the ingenious methods of self-care, and the incredible physical endurance of the Inuit hunters, who still fell prey to the bitter cold. He foresaw the need to study all these and other related problems of the Inuit "who are now subjected to abrupt changes…in their entire way of life."

He wrote about an old Inuk man from Arviat on Hudson Bay who suffered from advanced

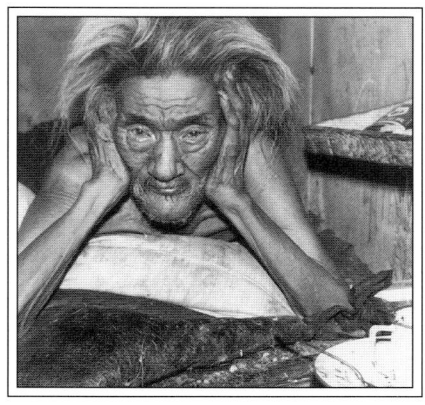

An elderly tuberculosis patient from Arviat who refused to be evacuated.

tuberculosis of the lungs and had passed on the disease to several grandchildren, who died of tuberculous meningitis. Otto had visited him several times in his home where he lay in a darkened corner, coughing up blood-tinged sputum. During each visit Otto explained that for the sake of all those in his community, he should go south for treatment. The old man refused every time. Finally one Tuesday, Otto made it clear that a plane was coming on Friday to take him south to hospital. On Thursday the old man died.

Otto noted that women were much more vulnerable to tuberculosis because of their sedentary lifestyle and the stress of repeated pregnancies. He described the devastation inflicted on the family when a wife and mother had to be flown south for prolonged treatment. Children had to be "farmed out" to friends and relatives, a disruptive and often traumatic experience. Left on their own, men tended to drift towards alcoholism or infidelity. A cure, however satisfying, of a tuberculous wife and mother was overshadowed by the ruinous social disruption of her family.

The trail-blazing 1959 article proved to be the turning point in Otto's career. Questions and comments came to him and to the Ottawa headquarters of the Department of National Health and Welfare from many points in North America and Europe. But one medical colleague was not impressed. Otto had met Dr. Jack Hildes on board the *C.D. Howe* after leaving Pangnirtung in September 1957. Both he and Otto had examined and treated patients at every port until the ship docked back in Montreal. At that time Hildes worked for the Defence Research Board; later, he became assistant professor of internal medicine at the University of Manitoba.

Otto handed his associate the article destined to be published in the CMAJ and asked for his opinion. Hildes was not a man to pussyfoot around: "You can do much better," he said. "All you've written is nothing more than a great pot-pourri of interesting things about the North. You've got enough material for ten articles. Why can't you be more focused?" In vain Otto tried to explain that the title was "Observations…" and he had intended the article as nothing more.

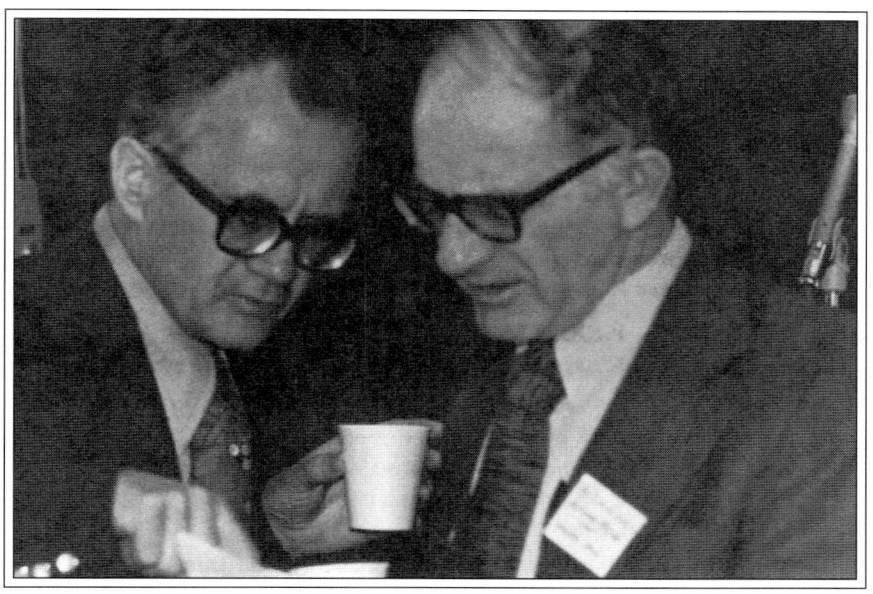

Otto Schaefer (left) and Jack Hildes (right) at the Churchill Health Conference in 1975.

The mutual irritation was exacerbated later when Hildes wrote a letter to the editor of the CMAJ, suggesting that the major push for health care studies in the North had come from the University of Manitoba. Otto replied, refuting the inaccurate claim. Hildes responded with a few sarcastic comments in a second letter.

But once those thorny patches were out of the way, the two became lifelong friends and enthusiastic collaborators in their research work. Otto did revise his article somewhat, following Hildes' suggestions, before sending it off. Later they would co-author several medical articles for publication.

It was an interesting partnership: the two men shared a tireless enthusiasm for subjects that captured their interest. After a hard day's work, they would often get together for two or three hours in the evening to discuss plans and projects. When energy started to fade, Hildes would mutter, "Aw, come on, Otto. Let's have another cup of coffee and keep working." Otto has always felt a sense of indebtedness to Jack Hildes for his help, advice and correction near the beginning of his career. He considered Hildes one of the finest clinicians he had ever met. Hildes, in turn, took great delight in being able to foster the work of a junior colleague whose talents he recognized early.

Hildes had wide interests and realized that many diseases had their origin in social problems. He was a leader in the field of adaptation studies, which included the Inuit adaptation to cold.

Some time later, Otto boasted to Jack Hildes that "I can eat anything that the Eskimos eat." Hildes stashed that comment away in his memory until the time came to put Otto to the test: "I've brought you a special treat, some nice fresh frozen meat," he said. Otto accepted the gift, and proceeded to eat it with zest. But it didn't taste so good, and he said as much to Hildes. Then he caught sight of the slightest smirky indrawing of his cheek, and knew that something was up. For a while Hildes just gazed at the ceiling, unconcerned. Then he thought he'd better come clean:

"You're always swaggering that you can eat anything, so I brought you this special walrus meat that I got from Eskimo friends at Igloolik. I'm sure you wouldn't mind me telling you that it had been lying in a hut for dog food for six years and that it had been thawed and frozen every year. But they said it was still good."

Otto gulped and suddenly didn't feel so well. Then he and Jack Hildes leaned back in their chairs and laughed. Henceforth he would keep his eclectic tastes for food to himself.

26
The Yukon

This is the law of the Yukon,
and ever she makes it plain:
Send not your foolish and feeble;
send me your strong and your sane.
Strong for the red rage of battle;
sane, for I harry them sore;
Sent me men girt for the combat,
men who are grit to the core...
Them will I take to my bosom,
them will I glut with my meat;
But the others—the misfits,
the failures—I trample under my feet.

Robert W. Service (1944:13)

THE Yukon has been called the last great wilderness region of North America. Occupying Canada's extreme northwest corner, it is a land of snowy mountains, white spruce and birch forests, fast-flowing rivers, Dall sheep, and grizzly bears. It is also a land of memories: memories of the gold strike in Bonanza Creek in 1896 that drew thousands to the shanty town of Dawson; memories of the glorious Klondike Days when the passion for gold brought luxury to the few and cruel hardship and suffering to the many.

Living at Aklavik in the Mackenzie Delta, Otto and Didi had often looked west and longed to visit the territory on the other side of the Richardson Mountains. Once they had flown to Old Crow in the remote far north of the Yukon to examine and treat patients. Now the

Department of Health and Welfare was posting them for two years to Whitehorse, capital of the Yukon, a town of about 7000 located 120 km north of the British Columbia border. In the summer of 1960, Otto was appointed chief of the medical staff of the new 100-bed hospital and Director of Indian and Inuit Health Care for the Yukon and northern British Columbia.

Otto admitted that Whitehorse "did not have the attraction of Baffin Island," probably because it was far too civilized and modern. Certainly here they would not have to melt river ice for drinking water and snow for washing. He anticipated it would be like a town in northern British Columbia, with good roads and modern amenities, and he proved to be right.

The two years in Whitehorse were a happy time for the family. On many wonderful family outings they struck out for the wilds to ski, hike, or fish. Nurse Shirley Donaghue remembers "a familiar sight around Whitehorse in those days was Didi and Otto riding their bikes with little ones on little bikes following up behind."

At that time most of the patients were Indians. The majority spoke English, and Otto had little difficulty relating to them. Iris Stout, who worked as a public health nurse, commented on "his genuine interest in the Indians, who seemed to appreciate his sincerity and responded well to him." But Otto found the Indians quite different from the Inuit. True, they seemed to be just as hardy and resourceful and supportive of one another, but he felt them to be somewhat aloof and at times resentful, as if they could not trust a white man.

Not all of his cases were Native people. In fact, one of the most baffling was that of a young Swiss trapper who came to the hospital with a high fever and prostration. On admission, the desperately ill young man fell under the care of a specialist in internal medicine from Vancouver, one of the short-term doctors on staff. The doctor did a thorough examination and ordered a series of tests, but found it impossible to determine what was wrong. He even made long-distance calls to Vancouver and Toronto, seeking help from senior consultants. At the end he was none the wiser. Two other doctors on the staff of the

Whitehorse hospital were just as baffled. In desperation, the visiting doctor started his patient on treatment for typhoid fever, one of the possible diagnoses. But the sick young man did not improve.

Otto and nurse Emmi Nemetz were doing ward rounds when the doctor from Vancouver called them aside. He had tried everything, he said, but the patient was going downhill and looked like he would not survive. Would Otto take a few minutes to have a look at him? Otto did so, and after a few minutes, shouted in the ear of the semiconscious patient: "Did you eat bear meat?" The young man said nothing. Otto tried the same question in French. Still no answer. Finally he repeated it in German. The patient still did not speak, but nodded his head just enough to give the answer they sought.

Immediately they estimated his weight and started him on the appropriate dose of the medicine for trichinosis, a disease caused by a parasite that infests polar bears and walruses. The Swiss trapper gradually improved and admitted he had eaten raw polar bear meat. Later Otto removed a small bit of muscle from the patient's lower leg; examination under a microscope confirmed the diagnosis he had suspected. Making the correct diagnosis was nothing to boast about, he said. He just happened to have seen a few cases of trichinosis while working at Aklavik.

If living was easier at Whitehorse, some problems were formidable. One in particular ruined his sleep at night and tore at this heart. He had never before seen such drunkenness. It was hard to miss it, especially during the evening supper hour when the bars were closed. Patrons staggered out onto the street, slobbering and swearing, and leaned against lamp posts or parked cars or anything, waiting until the bars re-opened. "Sometimes you could hardly walk down the street," said Iris Stout.

It was hard to sit back and ignore the problem, but it took one particular patient to spur Otto into action. A heartbroken Indian woman from the Teslin Lake area sobbed out her story of grief: within a single week she had lost her husband and son, both murdered in drunken fights outside a hotel pub at Johnson's Crossing at the north end of the lake. She blamed the white proprietor of the bar, who was known to willingly sell booze to people already staggering. Since the opening of the Alaska highway, that pub at Johnson's Crossing could be easily reached, and its influence had wrecked the lives of many in nearby Indian settlements.

Otto could have filled up a black book of tragedies, all alcohol-related. He had already seen newborn infants with brain damage, the so-called foetal alcohol syndrome. He saw firsthand how drinking white men took advantage of Native women.

He would never forget Sam Raddy, a tall Inuk from the Mackenzie Delta who lost his sight after drinking methyl alcohol while working on the DEW line. Sam's wife was one of five people who died following that binge. Having paid a monstrous price for his boozing, Sam was willing to talk to others in his community and beyond, hoping they would avoid such folly.

Statistics told the story: In the 1960s, 30 to 40 percent of the deaths caused by accidents and poisoning in Indians and Inuit of the Yukon and Northwest Territories were alcohol-related. As Otto wrote later in a medical journal: "Alcohol…has only intensified the degradation and frustration with their own [Native] social structure and now causes most of their health problems" (Schaefer, 1975a:101).

Otto knew it would be risky to campaign on behalf of the Native people against alcohol abuse. Hotels and pub-keepers were thriving on Native trade and hardly likely to co-operate. For another thing, he was told that "everyone drinks in the North," a statement not so far from the truth.

As an employee of National Health and Welfare, Otto got little encouragement from others in the Department. Furthermore, Fred Collins, the commissioner of the Yukon, objected to any sort of regulation or control: "We must not differentiate by races," he said. When some of the Indian communities wanted to be declared alcohol-free, Collins opposed their wishes with the argument "Then we'll have all kinds of smuggling." It was a tough battle, harder and more taxing than any of the hardships Otto had faced travelling by dog team. But halting the destruction caused by alcohol was a burden he was prepared to shoulder, whatever the opposition.

For a start, he and Flo Whyard, editor of the *Whitehorse Star*, founded the Indian Friendship Society and kept it going until Native people could take over. The society provided a valuable forum where the Indians could confront the alcohol problem head on and make their own decisions about controlling it. While no legislation came out of those sessions, the subject drew wide attention—a vital first step, in Otto's opinion.

Both in the *Whitehorse Star*, and later in Yellowknife's *News of the North*, Otto made strong statements like "alcohol is the greatest direct and indirect killer of Native people in the North" (Todd, 1982:A5). He led a campaign to close down some of the many bars in town, which brought him cold stares of resentment. He openly criticized the serving of alcohol by white pub-keepers to Indians who could hardly stand up. But he was careful enough to avoid mention of something that was common knowledge—that many pub-keepers had repeatedly cheated their Indian customers.

He talked on the radio, not limiting himself solely to the alcohol menace but also stressing the need for good health measures. He gave public addresses that were reported in the *Whitehorse Star*, the *Inuvik Drum* and the *Yukon News*. At times he felt like Don Quixote tilting at windmills. And he certainly won no popularity awards. But he could simply do no less.

27

On the Launching Pad

Back in Edmonton at the Camsell Hospital for Indians and Inuit during the summer of 1962, Otto would soon be facing the challenge of his life. He had served three two-year terms in the Western and Eastern Arctic and Yukon Territory and had gained experience that few others in his profession could match. He had shouldered what someone called an "overwhelming load" of acute and chronic diseases, scattered epidemics, and frequent accidents—all combined with public health work and frequent travels to outposts and settlements. In the realm of service, he had made what he called a reasonable contribution. Now he was ready for fresh fields of endeavour.

Otto had already made several trips to survey the Inuit population. In the summer of 1958 he had flown with a team from Edmonton to the Central Arctic to conduct health and nutrition surveys at Spence Bay, Coppermine, and Holman Island. While other members of the team were taking x-rays to screen for TB, he examined patients and recorded their state of health and general nutrition. From these studies, he developed a system for determining the health care needs of these three communities.

Motivated by what he described to me as "the appalling state of health of the Native population in the North," he determined to go beyond the treating of disease. The time had come to embark on a program of all-encompassing, systematic research. What were the causes of and factors contributing to the widespread illness and disease?

Otto's first article about health in the Arctic, published in the *Canadian Medical Association Journal* in 1959, had evoked far more interest than either he or Jack Hildes could have imagined. A flood of letters had poured into the Headquarters of the Department of Health and Welfare in Ottawa. Dr. Harry Procter, Assistant Director of Indian and Eskimo Health Services, having perused most of the letters, decided that they should not pile up any longer. He phoned Otto in Edmonton:

"For quite a while I've been accumulating a stack of letters from medical scientists from all over North America and Europe. They've read your article and want to know more about health care in the Arctic," he said. "To be honest, I've reached my limit in trying to reply. When can you answer them? I know I can't cope with all the questions."

"Neither can I," said Otto. "It's a while since that article came out, and things have been changing so rapidly that much of what I wrote is out of date. As you know, the DEW line has made tremendous changes in the North."

"So what do you propose?" asked Dr. Procter.

"I would like to go back to the Arctic and conduct more studies and surveys, and compare the results with previous findings. It would be interesting as well to compare results in various locations. But of course I can't do that and keep on with my regular work at the Camsell," he said.

The whole issue was left in abeyance, and for a while Otto just carried on at the Camsell. A few months later he received from Dr. Procter the letter that would determine his career for the next thirty years. The Department of Indian and Eskimo Health Services would create a special Northern Medical Research Unit. Would Otto be willing to serve as its first director?

Otto conferred with Didi, always his partner in decision making. It would mean flying the length and breadth of the Arctic, away from his family, for two-month periods in spring and summer, to say nothing of short winter trips and emergency work. The Department might supply a secretary; otherwise, he would be on his own.

It was a daunting proposition, as are most pioneering and trail-blazing ventures. Otto had already expressed his interest and had offered himself, but could not shake off feelings of inadequacy. The extra burden for Didi was another concern he could not easily cast aside. It was adventurous Didi who finally gave him the push he needed to tell Dr.

Procter that he would take on the job. Early in 1964, Otto became the first director of the Northern Medical Research Unit.

28
The Changing North

Few peoples have ever experienced such drastic changes in their way of living and dying as did the Eskimos and Indians in the Canadian North. (Schaefer, 1973: 196)

BEFORE the early 1950s, most Canadian Inuit lived in hunting camps or settlements as large family groups. They enjoyed a nomadic life, moving their sealskin tents to the rhythm of the seasons or the unpredictable migrations of sea mammals, fish, and caribou. Igloos were used primarily by men on hunting trips.

Inuit on the coastal areas of Greenland and Alaska had been reached by explorers, whalers, trappers, and prospectors from the late eighteenth century onward. Some Canadian Inuit, by way of contrast, had had little or no contact with white men until World War II, when the skies began to buzz with airplanes and radio signals. In less than a generation, an "invasion" by the affluent civilization of modern Western man would change the world of the Canadian Inuit forever.

Some of the changes were beneficial. Never again would the Inuit be threatened by the recurrent famines of the old days, which wiped out entire settlements. New weapons made for better hunting, and new food staples kept them going when game was scarce. Never again would tuberculosis be allowed to run rampant, disabling and destroying young and old alike. Never again would a typhoid epidemic be allowed to take the lives of 12 percent of the population, as happened in Cumberland Sound in 1940 (Schaefer, 1975a).

The old order was dying. Otto, for one, regretted its demise. In the *University of Manitoba Medical Journal* he wrote:

> *Where formerly one heard the melancholy howling of sled dogs to majestic curtains of Northern lights moving across the star-studded sky, your ears are now insulted by screaming skidoos racing along neon-lighted streets; and where you saw hunters bringing seals, fish or caribou home and women scraping skins and sewing warm fur clothing, you now see them buying parkas made in Montreal or Winnipeg; and where you heard the beat and ay-ay-yah refrain of a drum dance, you hear now the bang-bang-bang of the latest gangster movie or the noisy and violent fights in front of the beer parlour.*
> (Schaefer, 1975a:98)

Before 1955, the pace of change was not too disruptive. But the building of the DEW line radar installations all across the North accelerated the whole process. A string of military and civilian airports brought remote areas out of their isolation. Hired to help with the construction of the DEW line stations, many Inuit left the traditional life and began to live like white people. Most needed little enticement to leave their old ways.

To create communities for year-round living at various centres, the Department of Northern Affairs erected houses and schools, aiming for 100 percent literacy in English. The majority of Eastern Arctic Inuit were already able to read and write letters in Inuktitut syllabic script. Working at the defence installations, the erstwhile hunters of the family ate their meals at the cafeteria. With the money they earned and a generous government grant, many would soon move to houses with oil heat and electricity. They could buy clothes and food from a government-sponsored store or the Hudson's Bay Company outlet. The women no longer had to sew clothing or scrounge for food. The upheaval happened so quickly that it was like being catapulted into modern civilization. And it made for profound changes in the social life and environment. Even more important were the changes in the personal values and attitudes, family structure, and overall culture of the Inuit.

In his new job, Otto would focus on how the drastic changes in lifestyle had affected the health and nutrition of the Inuit. But he would also be studying and recording the impact of the intruding civilization on their way of living. He had no illusions about the size and difficulty of his task. Medical research on a small, compact population is one thing: it's quite another to travel over great distances using uncertain methods of communication to study small, isolated groups of people. In the Northwest Territories, for example, fewer than 50,000 people occupied more than 2.5 million km², an area comparable to the land mass of India. But it would be a wonderful opportunity to study and compare isolated groups of people, some still living traditional lives and others already "acculturated" to Western living. Recording the changes in the health of the Native population under this influence should be a great boon to future health care planning, he thought, and would perhaps provide clues to the causes of certain "diseases of civilization."

29

Surveys Across the North

It was 1:30 a.m. on April 12, 1964 when Otto Schaefer finally put down his pen and stethoscope. A school served as his clinic at Gjoa Haven on King William Island, just off the northern coast of mainland Canada. While other team members were x-raying the residents to exclude TB, Otto had examined 124 people, recorded his findings in a book, and taken photographs.

He walked outside for a breath of fresh air. The sun was just sinking below the horizon. The Central Arctic Survey was into its third week, but his mind was on other things. Looking north over the flat, featureless island, he thought of the terrible tragedy that had taken place on these barren wastes 117 years before. The British navigator-explorer Sir John Franklin, in search of the Northwest Passage to the Orient, had come within 150 km of the route that would have led him to ultimate success. Unfortunately, he then tried to sail through the ice floes of Victoria Strait to the west of King William Island. There, both his ships, the *Erebus* and the *Terror*, became locked in the ice (Struzik, 1991:14). In June 1847, near Victory Point at the north end of the island, Franklin fell ill and died. Soon after his death, one ship sank and the other was dashed against the rocks by moving ice.

Captain Frances Crozier was left to lead the remaining 105 men of Franklin's expedition. Towing their supplies on heavy sleds, they set off on foot, heading south. They must have trudged close to the spot where Otto was standing, he reasoned, on their hopeless trek toward the mainland and the mouth of the Great Fish (later, the Back) River where they hoped to get help from Hudson's Bay Company traders. As the short Arctic summer waned and their supplies ran out, they fell one by one. From the trail of bones, tin cans, and other relics, searchers later traced their path down to the Adelaide Peninsula, where even the hardiest survivors finally gave up.

Otto thought it ironic that Gjoa Haven acquired its name not from the Franklin debacle, but from one of the few success stories to emerge from the quest for the Northwest Passage. Roald Amundsen, the great Norwegian explorer and the first man to successfully navigate the Passage, spent the winter there in 1903–04. He named the place "Gjoa Haven" after his ship, the *Gjoa* (Pool, 1988).

Otto would embark upon two Arctic surveys in 1964 in his role as director of the Northern Medical Research Unit: a one-month Central Arctic Survey in the spring and another month with the Eastern Arctic Patrol in the fall, on board the *C.D. Howe*. Having done similar studies in both areas a few years before, he looked forward to comparing his old findings with the new. But he also hoped that these two surveys would provide orientation for future field studies to investigate specific health problems, such as the causes of infant mortality.

Each patient could expect to get three types of service: a detailed interview in his or her own language, a thorough physical examination, and one or more tests—such as blood and urine examinations—to exclude certain infectious and metabolic diseases. If a patient suffered from any illness, Otto would do his best to offer the necessary treatment. A patient could also expect to be asked apparently nonmedical questions: How many caribou did you get last winter? How much fishing did you do? How long did the supply last? How much food did you buy from the Hudson's Bay store?

Leaving from Edmonton in April 1964 in a single-engine Norseman plane, Otto travelled with the x-ray team of three people to several locations along the shore of mainland Canada, ending up at Pelly Bay at the north end of the Keewatin District. The team members took along their own food and shared the cooking duties for the infrequent times when local people did not welcome them into their homes. Otto even took along his dental equipment, priding himself that he could do painless extractions. In fact, his friend Canon Webster from Coppermine (a sort of amateur dentist) had shown him how to fill cavities in teeth.

Years later, on a return visit, Otto felt rather pleased to see some of his old fillings still in place.

The team had a busy time in Coppermine examining, treating, and x-raying 357 patients in just three days. Otto was glad to hear good reports from the two nurses stationed there and to see so many healthy children. Seven years before, he had flown to Coppermine on an emergency call. A nurse had radioed for help after an outbreak of measles with life-threatening pneumonia. Otto had arrived to find the school closed and the small nursing station jammed full of children on stretchers and mats on the floor. Wheezing, feverish children had been brought in from a number of camps, including nearby Rae River. It must have been a nightmarish experience. But Otto had taken along a good supply of broad-spectrum antibiotics specific for the secondary chest complications. Fortunately the children recovered. Questioned about any recurrence of measles epidemics since 1957, the nurse shook her head. The credit must go to the measles vaccine, she said.

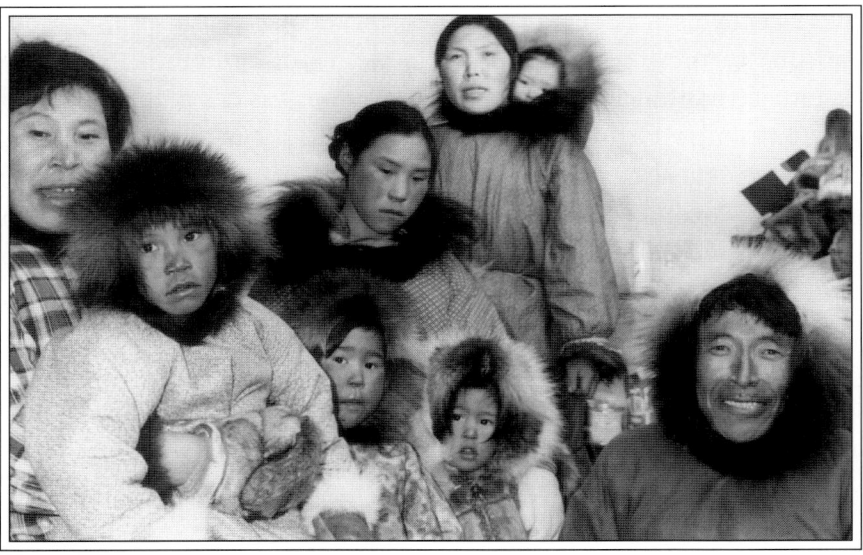

A family from the area between Coppermine and Bathurst Inlet, awaiting medical examination.

While working at Coppermine in 1964, Otto received a call about an emergency even more serious than the measles outbreak seven years before. An epidemic of meningitis was raging in the Keewatin District, west of Hudson Bay. He immediately set aside his survey timetable. Dr. Gordon Butler, regional director for Health and Welfare, asked him to take off as soon as he could for Baker Lake and Arviat.

Otto had seen his first case of meningitis in 1956, when a family arrived in Pangnirtung with an 18-month-old child in a critical state. They had travelled for a whole week from Hoare Bay over the mountains and on the last day spent anxious hours on a drifting ice floe on Cumberland Sound. Sadly, Otto could do nothing to save the child. A vicious and often fatal disease, meningitis attacked children in the Arctic at least fifty times more often than elsewhere in Canada. In some cases it struck as a complication of tuberculosis; in others, it was caused by the same bacteria responsible for pneumonia. If the children survived the initial onslaught, they were often left with serious disabilities affecting their nervous system. It was meningitis in early childhood that left the celebrated Helen Keller deaf and blind.

Knowing that the University of Manitoba had some responsibility for the health care in this area, Dr. Butler had already contacted Dr. Jack Hildes. Otto looked forward to collaborating once again with his old friend from Winnipeg. Dr. A.R. Ronald, a microbiologist, would be going along on the emergency flight.

At Arviat, Baker Lake, and Rankin Inlet, they quickly learned that the seriousness of the epidemic had not been exaggerated. Some children had already succumbed. Others lay prostrate with high fever, headache, and vomiting. Some had convulsions similar to those of grand mal epilepsy. Otto recognized that those children in the advanced stages—with shock, cold and clammy limbs, and deep coma—were beyond hope. Yet many others could be saved. Dr. Ronald took swabs from the throats of nearly all the children and found the offending bacteria in most cases to be *Hemophilus influenzae*. Otto and Jack Hildes performed spinal taps to be sure of the diagnosis of meningitis. They gave the children the appropriate antibiotic, which reversed the course of the disease in many cases.

Treatment of the established disease was clearly of vital importance, but for Otto it was not enough. Why were these children so vulnerable? Exposure to cold was undoubtedly a factor, but there must be others. Dr. Butler blamed poor housing. Surprisingly, Otto found that Inuit children from warm, oil-heated homes were hit with the disease far more often than those living in sealskin tents. He concluded that poor humidification of the comfortable houses caused the lining of the throat to dry out and crack, thereby allowing a point of entry for the bacteria. The same dryness had been the cause of the common nosebleeds in children living in the residential school in Aklavik. In both circumstances, Otto found children who breathed through the mouth (because of enlarged adenoids, etc.) were more susceptible. Not until the 1980s would a vaccine, given early in infancy, protect a child against this type of meningitis, caused by *Hemophilus influenzae* (although a vaccine against meningococcal meningitis would be developed in the 1960s). For the immediate future, the simple expedient of moistening the air children breathed could sharply reduce the incidence of the disease in the Arctic.

On board the *C.D. Howe* in September 1964, at the conclusion of the Eastern Arctic Patrol, Otto wrote his usual comprehensive report. He started by saying "The medical picture has changed remarkably during the eleven years I have had occasion to observe it in the Western, Central and Eastern Arctic" (Schaefer, 1964:8). Some of the changes were impressively for the better. The sharp reduction in the incidence of active cases of tuberculosis he attributed to extensive case finding and effective anti-TB treatment. In fact, for five years no Natives had died from TB, once the North's terrible scourge. But he was concerned about the large numbers of women and children suffering from anaemia. Further, in a number of people he had found diabetes, a disease previously unreported in the North. He also wanted to investigate the families of several women who had retained placentas after childbirth, two of whom had died as a result.

Most of all, Otto suspected that the social and economic changes that had overtaken the Inuit were having a bad effect on their nutrition and general health. He thought that this subject deserved to be singled out and studied intensively. By comparing the eating habits and activities of residents in various communities affected to a greater or lesser degree by these major changes, he hoped to find the answers.

30
The Executioners

IN 1966, Otto found himself in the midst of a murder trial in Spence Bay. It was a strange place for the Canadian legal system to dispense justice. In the schoolroom reserved for the occasion, the walls were lined with coloured poster cutouts that the children had made the week before. Elderly Judge John Sissons, veteran jurist of the Northwest Territories, presided at the teacher's desk. Dressed in black gowns and crisp, white collar tabs, lawyers for the defence and prosecution sat before him, rising to their feet periodically to address the court.

The jury—three local Inuit and three white people—sat in an enclave by themselves, as if a little distance from the rest might help objectivity. At the very back of the classroom sat a large group of Inuit spectators, silent and impassive. Most of the space between them and the front was filled with witnesses, reporters, and court stenographers.

The two accused young men seemed like minor characters in the drama. They looked out of place and remarkably boyish, as though they had only recently left the classroom. Shooyook and his cousin Aiyaoot, both about 20 years old, were being tried for murdering Aiyaoot's mother, Soosee. Yet they seemed unconcerned as they sat side by side, saying nothing. They occasionally smiled but mostly kept their eyes lowered to the floor.

The facts of the case were clear, said Mr. David Searle, counsel for the Crown, in his opening remarks. The charge read that on July 15, 1965 near isolated Fort Ross (about 320 km north of Spence Bay) the two accused had "jointly committed the capital murder of Soosee." They had freely admitted to shooting her. What's more, it was common knowledge that Soosee's husband had encouraged them to do it. Amazingly, Shooyook's father had written down the details in his diary and presented his report to the RCMP.

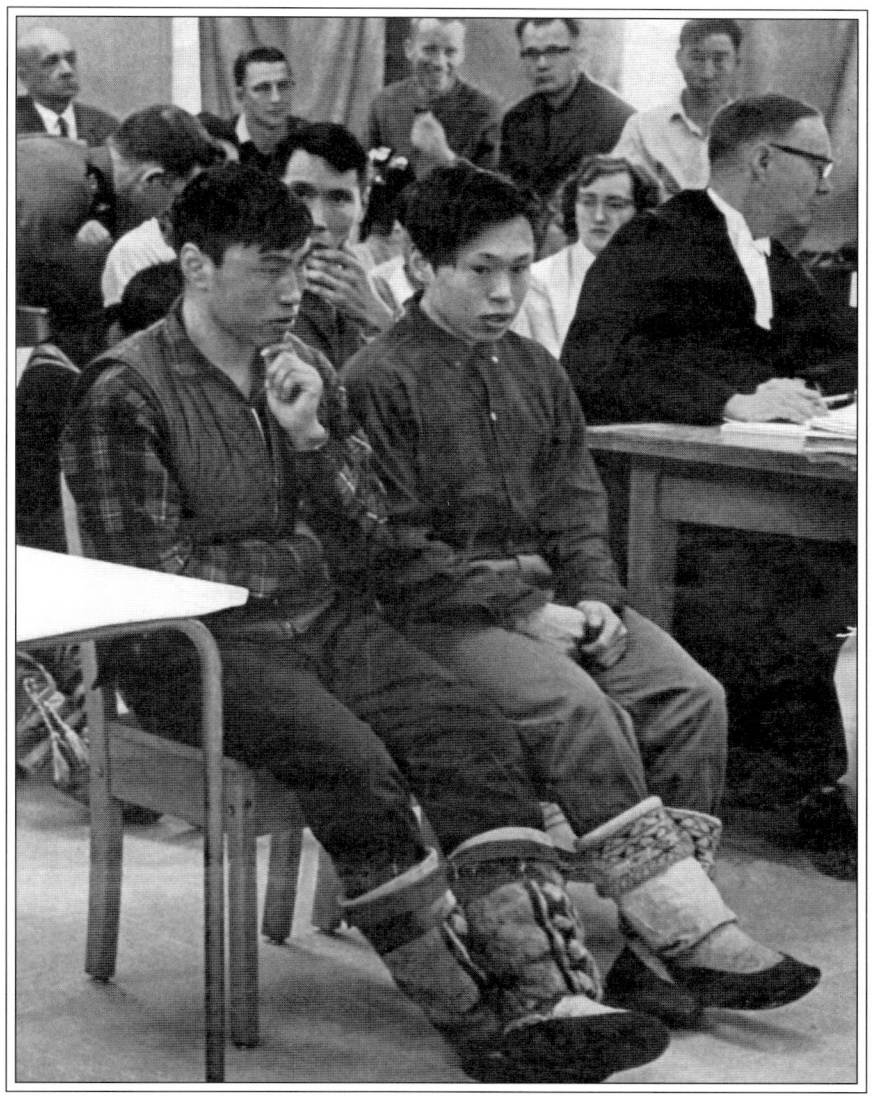

Aiyaoot and Shooyook on trial for murder in Spence Bay in April 1966. Photo by Farley Mowat.

Absolutely no one had lamented the demise of Soosee. Born in 1915, she had suffered from schizophrenia as a young woman and created

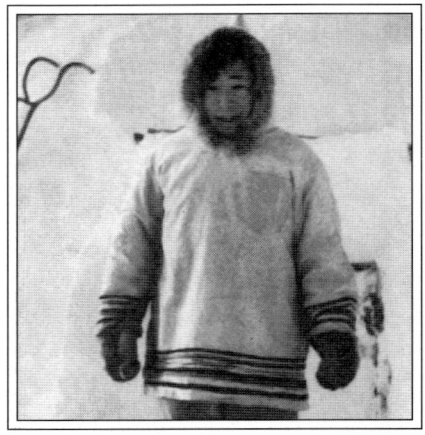

Soosee, who was put to death by her son Aiyaoot and nephew Shooyook. Photo by Farley Mowat.

havoc for her family and the Fort Ross community. She had visual hallucinations and paranoia, suspecting that people were out to get her. When she became violent and a menace to her children, two men had set out on the long journey by dog team for the RCMP detachment at Spence Bay. An RCMP aircraft subsequently landed at Fort Ross and flew Soosee to Spence Bay, whence she eventually reached the Charles Camsell Hospital in Edmonton. There she was seen by a consultant psychiatrist, who denied there was any evidence of schizophrenia, labelled her condition as "acute anxiety state," and sent her home without specific treatment.

Five years later, in 1964, she was on the rampage again, this time threatening to kill all the children in the camp. All winter long her husband didn't dare leave her behind in their igloo. Unable to hunt, with food supplies running low and everyone haggard from sleeplessness, he asked his neighbours to contact the RCMP again. This time Otto Schaefer was working at Spence Bay and took it upon himself to examine Soosee. Confident that the diagnosis of schizophrenia was correct, he wrote a letter to accompany her to the Alberta Mental Hospital near Edmonton. Like a cornered wildcat, she flew at the attendants on arrival and had to be placed in a straitjacket. Yet after four months under treatment, she had improved enough to be returned home.

It wasn't long until the whole community was fleeing in terror from the tall, husky, demented woman. In a fit of violence she smashed and broke the arm of her own baby. She slashed the family's summertime sealskin tent with a knife, leaving it in shreds. Even more than her violent behaviour, others feared evil spells and curses: she threatened to "breathe the devil" on them. Almost everyone moved away from the settlement for a while, hoping the solitude would quiet her down. They paddled in boats to a small nearby island where they could keep a watch on her through the telescopes they used for hunting.

After three days of watching her rampaging through the camp in an orgy of destruction, the group decided to act. Soosee's husband, Napachee-Kadlac, instructed Shooyook and Aiyaoot to return to their camp and try to save what was

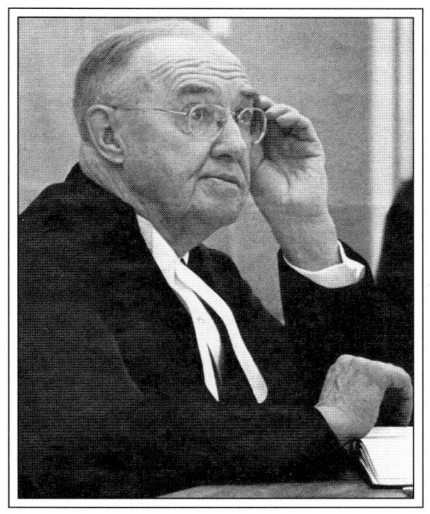

Justice John Sissons. Photo by Farley Mowat.

left. If they found Soosee as mad and violent as ever, they were to shoot her. Through the telescope, the distraught husband watched the two armed men approach the camp. He saw Soosee suddenly run out towards them, screaming and swinging a rifle. Then he heard four shots and it was all over.

Peace and calm reigned at last in the small Fort Ross settlement. The outcome was accepted by all, including Shooyook and Aiyaoot, who saw no reason to hide. In fact, three months later they travelled to Spence Bay to trade. There Shooyook was arrested, flown to Yellowknife, and charged with capital murder.

As the trial proceeded, it became clear that this was far from being the usual contest between prosecution and defence. In his remarks to the jury, Judge Sissons summed up the feelings of many when he said: "This is a difficult case. Our sympathy must be with these people who found themselves in this impossible situation...I do not envy you your task." Before the trial, several of the white people at Spence Bay had already prejudged the case, declaring that not only must the two accused be found guilty and punished, but Napachee-Kadlac should not get off the hook. After all, he had put them up to it. There was yet another strange twist: all the Inuit witnesses were called by the prosecution. They had nothing to hide. Napachee-Kadlac freely admitted that he was the one who had instructed the two to shoot Soosee if they had to.

Most telling of all was the diary of Kadloo, father of Shooyook. Reading from syllabic script on yellowed, tattered slips of paper, he described in detail Soosee's mounting rages and the fear that she could breathe her madness onto others. Twice they had tied her up, and each time she had broken the tough sealskin bonds—a sign of supernatural strength, they thought. Kadloo described what he had seen through his telescope as the two accused approached Soosee, rifles at the ready.

Two of the defence witnesses were Dr. A.D. MacPherson and Dr. Keith A. Yonge, psychiatrists from Edmonton. Both had examined Soosee, but they had different opinions. One confidently stated that she had suffered from paranoid schizophrenia, a serious mental disorder often accompanied by violence. The other claimed she had been mentally deranged, but "definitely not schizophrenic." As the third witness for the defence, Otto Schaefer described the condition in which he had found Soosee in 1964. He testified that he had ordered that she be evacuated to a mental hospital near Edmonton for treatment of schizophrenia and that she be kept there. Read to the court, his letter giving that order was deemed a mainstay for the argument of the defence.

Questioned by defence counsel William Morrow, Otto had further comments based on his broad knowledge of the North. In his experience, Inuit were terrified by abnormal behaviour, which they often attributed to evil spirits like those believed to be possessing the unfortunate Soosee. He said that Napachee-Kadlac deserved no blame for instigating the shooting, since "even primitive societies have a division of executive and legislative powers."

In a society where survival is a constant struggle, the welfare of the individual must take a back seat to that of the group, he testified. The Inuit people had time-tested ways of preserving the community against threats to its survival. The small group at Fort Ross, lacking a police force, mental hospitals, and all other facilities, had done their best to cope with a situation that endangered them all.

The jury retired and did not return with a decision for three hours. Before delivering the verdict, the foreman announced how difficult it had been, primarily because "we considered the Eskimos' culture as it affects the case." They found Aiyaoot not guilty and Shooyook guilty of manslaughter, adding a strong plea for leniency. Judge Sissons gave Shooyook a year's suspended sentence.

Some considered the whole trial an affront to the Inuit culture. Cameron Smith, a reporter from the Toronto *Globe and Mail*, wrote a long article entitled "The Law and the North: Is Canadian justice an injustice to the Eskimo?" (June 24, 1966:7). Even more scathing criticism came from an article by well-known author Farley Mowat, writing in *Maclean's* magazine. His article, entitled "The Executioners," denounced the entire proceedings. He used phrases like "the slow humiliation of a proud and self-reliant people," and asked, "Were these two men the real executioners—or were we all on trial?" (Mowat, 1966:7).

Farley Mowat's indictment lost a fair bit of its credibility, however, when *Maclean's* published a rebuttal to his charges written by L.A. Learmonth, a 46-year veteran of the North. Learmonth began by "pointing out a few of the many errors and the general falseness of Mowat's article" and then went on to cite specific details (Learmonth, 1966:31).

After a personal encounter with Mowat at Spence Bay a day or so after the trial, Otto Schaefer also felt disinclined to accept his passionate claims. Mowat had heard that a plane would be arriving in two days to transport Otto, the x-ray team, and a couple of patients to Cambridge Bay. He came to the nursing station where Otto was working and demanded that he be given a seat on that plane. Mowat's angry outburst when Otto told him the plane would be full and he could not dislodge any patient undermined the credibility of his written defence of the rights and dignity of the Inuit.

Was justice seen and done? Had the Canadian legal system shown respect for the Inuit society and acted to preserve the dignity of "the people par excellence," as Judge Sissons described them (Sissons, 1968:190)? Or had the *kadluna* (foreigners) and their laws run roughshod over a proud and self-reliant people, as Mowat contended? Otto believed the former. After all, a murder had been committed, whatever the circumstances, and could not be ignored. But he also believed that the court had shown respect for the culture of an isolated, aboriginal society seeking—without any outside help—to find a just and honourable solution to a crisis that threatened to wreck the community.

31
Human Adaptation

HUMAN beings have lived in the Arctic for more than 4000 years. The Inuit of Canada and their counterparts in Alaska, Siberia, and Greenland exhibit remarkable similarities of language, culture and art. For reasons which we Southerners may never comprehend, these circumpolar peoples chose to make the Arctic their home and began adjusting to its extraordinary rigours in order to survive. How successful had they been in adapting? What means had they found to protect themselves from the many dangers constantly threatening their lives?

Otto had seen plenty of tragedies. He would never forget one young man he had treated for frostbite and gangrene after his sled slipped off an ice floe and flung him into the frigid water. When Etuangat told Otto about his brother who went out hunting and never came back, he seemed to be saying that death was never far away. Yet for all the tragic stories, there were far more—if somewhat less dramatic—tales of successful living in an unforgiving environment.

Had Northerners' bodies undergone any changes to adapt to the cold, the food, and the constant challenge of harsh surroundings? What had the small clusters and settlements done to ensure survival? Otto Schaefer and Jack Hildes knew some of the answers, but they were determined to find out more. They planned a research project as part of the International Biology Program that was studying human adaptation. Similar studies had been going on in Iceland, Siberia, and northern Scandinavia. Hildes directed the Canadian component of the program, with Otto serving as "assistant and colleague."

They chose to survey two contrasting communities located not far apart on Melville Peninsula, north of Hudson Bay. Igloolik remained traditional, while Hall Beach had become more acculturated to modern

Canada. The two men spent several periods in winter and spring examining all the residents. A comparable study was then undertaken using inhabitants of Arctic Bay, on north Baffin Island, and Inuvik, in the Mackenzie Delta.

How does the human body react to cold? Hildes, a physiologist, had previously learned that the hands of the Inuit get some protection from the cold through improved peripheral circulation to the fingers. Hildes and Schaefer made interesting discoveries about sweating: the Inuit sweat more in the face, the only unclothed body part, but very little elsewhere, especially in the vulnerable hands and feet (Schaefer et al., 1974). The loss of heat from body extremities in sweat-soaked clothing could be critical in a cold environment. The investigators found the same sweating pattern existed in Inuit who had worked for many years in heated buildings, which suggested an inherited adaptation.

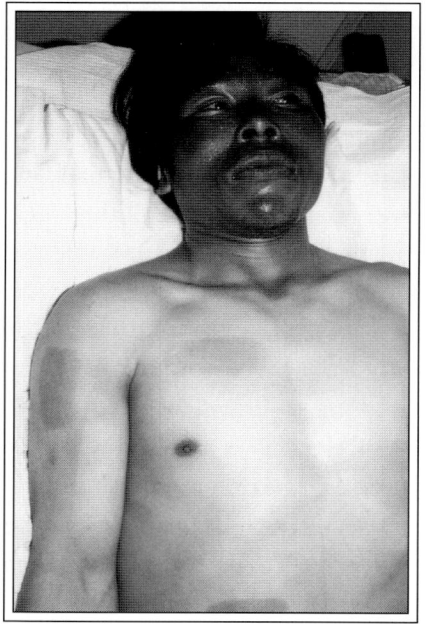

A resident of Igloolik taking part in the sweating test conducted by Otto Schaefer and Jack Hildes.

But these minor physiological adaptations could hardly be compared with the sophisticated adaptation to the cold of Arctic mammals like the caribou and polar bear. Each hair of the caribou hide is hollow, with a central core of the most effective insulator, air. Between the longer hairs are short wool-like hairs. The polar bear's protective layers of fat and thick fur that is impervious to water allow it to swim for long periods in icy water.

Certainly the human body's adaptation to cold would do little to protect a person from freezing to death. Far more important were the fur clothing that provided effective body insulation, the moss-insulated sealskin tents, and the simple but ingenious igloo.

Yet in spite of some obvious successes against the biting cold in most areas, a distressing failure remained. At Coppermine Otto had examined a 62-year-old man in the last stages of his life. Wasted in his limbs and gasping for breath, he sat up in bed barely able to speak. His lips and fingernails were blue. Yet he hadn't had a heart attack or pneumonia and had been active all his life—perhaps too active. Like countless others, he suffered, and soon died, from a condition called "Eskimo lung" or "frozen lung" (Schaefer et al., 1980a). It hit the most important members of the community, the hunters. Those who hunted often in the bitter winter cold suffered the most. Many could recall their trouble starting after they "froze their lungs" during a hectic time, often running in pursuit of game. Otto thought that deep and rapid breathing of cold air through the open mouth was the cause.

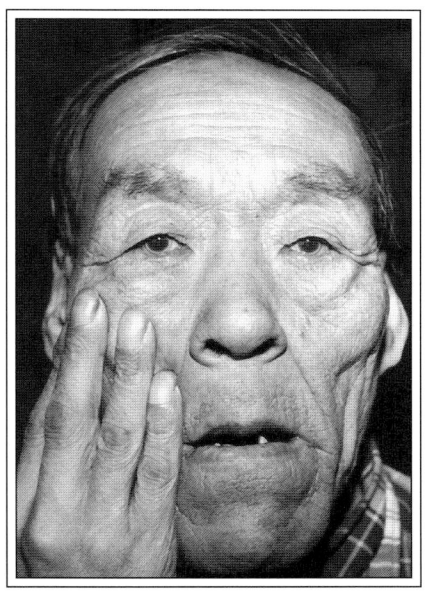

An elderly hunter from Igloolik with clubbing of the ends of his fingers caused by "frozen lung."

In Arctic Bay, where the traditional lifestyle prevailed, Hildes and Schaefer found the young men under age 25 to have good, healthy lungs, even though some of them smoked. But those over 40 showed evidence of lung damage, often severe, with consequent strain on the heart. By way of contrast, in Inuvik, an urbanized centre, the lungs of older men remained normal, except for those of Inuit and white trappers over 60 who had run fox traplines in their younger days.

The results of their study, published in the *Canadian Medical Association Journal* (Schaefer et al., 1980a), immediately stirred up controversy. Some said that cold air can't possibly damage the lungs because it is warmed and moistened in the nose and throat; dogs given an anaesthetic and then made to breathe cold air did not suffer any lung damage. But Hildes and Schaefer received support from Russian investigators, who reported that horses and dogs severely exercised in extreme winter conditions in Siberia also suffered damage to the lungs.

In their studies of adaptation of the human body, Hildes and Schaefer came across interesting deviations from the "normal" physiology. They found that the enlarged livers of many meat-eating Inuit could be explained by the body's need for more carbohydrates, which the liver can produce by converting proteins. As expected in people whose diet is mostly protein, their digestive system showed an inability to cope with starches and sugars. This sometimes led to a false diagnosis of diabetes (Schaefer, 1968). Otto also demonstrated that the Indians and Inuit are slow to metabolize alcohol and therefore cannot handle it as well as Caucasians (Fenna et al., 1971).

Other studies explained the Inuit susceptibility to viral epidemics and chronic infections like tuberculosis. The main defence against such assaults to health rests with the lymphocytes, which provide cellular immunity against these chronic diseases; for reasons which remain unclear, the lymphocytes in the bloodstream of Indians and Inuit performed poorly.

In his studies of Inuit adaptation to the cruel climate and hard living in the Arctic, Otto was impressed most of all by the social adjustment. He was struck by the extreme tolerance and the suppression of anger and hostility within the extended family. The autonomy of individuals was respected, provided they did not transgress the limits set to maintain the welfare and the integrity of the family. This social strategy encompassed the universally accepted need and desire to share with others. Far from perfect, and undoubtedly conditioned by the unique environment and the struggle to survive, the Inuit social structure made for the wholesome growth and development of individual family members.

The resourceful Inuit had shown they could adapt to Nature's most unforgiving conditions. But sadly, rapid, overwhelming changes brought by the "invasion" from the south would stretch their capacity for adaptation beyond its limits—and tear apart their social fabric.

32
Nutrition and Malnutrition

OTTO had always tried to maintain a healthful lifestyle, in spite of his busy schedule and other pressures. He and Didi kept themselves fit and active and encouraged all their children to enjoy the outdoor life. The whole family loved mountains, but it was not enough to simply gaze at their beauty and inhale the fresh, pine-scented mountain air. They liked to hike through the forests and climb the rocky slopes.

Skiing was a passion. Dr. Buzz Edwards of the University Hospital recalls attending a medical conference with Otto and skiing with him later. After a full day on the slopes, the two men relaxed in the warm, moist heat of a sauna, but Buzz refused to join Otto outside afterwards "for a roll in the snow with just our shorts on."

Otto was well known for his complete indifference to the food he ate. That indifference was all Jack Hildes had needed to trick him into eating the old dog food. But Otto was certainly interested in the diet and nutrition of his Inuit friends, a subject that occupied many hours of study and deep concern.

In 1965, as director of the Northern Medical Research Unit, Otto set up an ambitious program that grew out of the 1964 Central and Eastern Arctic Surveys. He described his self-imposed mandate as "the systematic examinations of health and nutrition status of several groups of Canadian Inuit populations and evaluation of the influence of documented changes in lifestyle and nutrition on their growth and physical as well as mental and social health."

He planned to carry out a questionnaire survey of food habits and activity in four diverse Inuit communities. He would contact personally as many individuals as he could, but would also rely on the help of nurses, missionaries, policemen, and teachers. He hoped to spend most of April and May at Holman Island and Coppermine, and devote June and July to Frobisher Bay (now Iqaluit) and Pangnirtung (Schaefer, 1965).

Otto looked forward to comparing and contrasting the four locations, all of which were at different stages of acculturation. The residents of Holman Island had been less influenced by the DEW line and other intrusions and still survived mainly from hunting and fishing. Coppermine people had previously relied on caribou, but since the migration of the great herds had become erratic, they had turned towards food sold by the Hudson's Bay Company or government-sponsored stores. Iqaluit, where more Inuit had settled than in any other community, was a good example of a wage-employment and store-food community. He expected to find a society unhealthy in more ways than one. He knew that the Pangnirtung of old had survived mainly by fishing and hunting, but had it too changed?

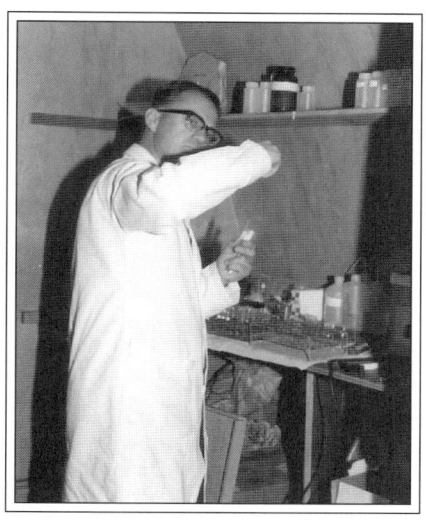

Dr. Schaefer's "lab" in the broom closet of the school at Holman Island during the community survey examinations done in March and April 1965.

He found the Holman Island people to be the healthiest of any in the Amundsen Gulf-Coppermine area. Although they had been buying more store food than previously with the extra income from higher-priced seal skins, few were obese and most were fit and active. The Coppermine people depended heavily on store food, mostly in the form of carbohydrates, both unrefined (flour and cereals) and refined (sugar). With the rapid growth in population and urbanization in Iqaluit, Native food sources had become totally inadequate, and store-bought food abounded. Alcohol consumption had skyrocketed.

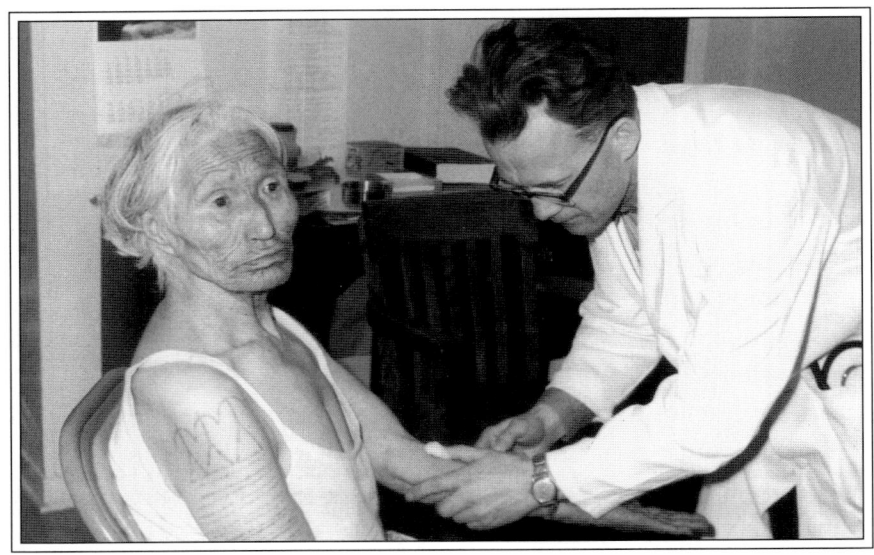

Dr. Schaefer taking a blood sample from an elderly resident of Coppermine.

Pangnirtung and the Cumberland Sound settlements were remarkably healthy in every sense, a finding that pleased Otto greatly. It was his first return visit after a long absence of eight years, and he regretted that Didi could not be there to share the joy he felt at being back at the place they called "paradise." He could not have had a warmer welcome from Etuangat and Nukinga, Amosie, and Paulusie, who all received him like a brother. Rosie, who had been Didi's domestic helper, insisted that he stay with her family. In a sense, it was like being home again.

The snow-capped mountains and the great fjord with its massive, sheer cliffs spoke to him of the eternal, the unchanging. But so much else had changed. The population of Pangnirtung itself had increased to about 200. The hospital had been closed and the building converted to an old folks' home. A nursing station functioned well under the care of the daughter of the respected Anglican missionary, Canon Arthur Turner. As the rapid development of Iqaluit included a large airport, doctors could now fly out twice a month and attend to the needs of the sick in a couple of days.

Otto looked around for the little white house that for his family had been a home no other could match. But it had been moved away, and was now occupied by a family on welfare. A nice pan-abode house (prefabricated house of simulated logs) had been built for Otto's successor, but of course there was no doctor now. The area around the site of his old home—once described by Didi as "our beautiful meadows"—had been levelled off to make a landing strip.

Etuangat, now 65, insisted on accompanying Otto on his survey trips to all the camps on Cumberland Sound. This time they travelled together by motorboat. Etuangat said that not many sled dogs remained: the efficient but noisy snowmobile had displaced them. Times had indeed changed!

The DEW line installations on Baffin Island were slowly being downsized, but some Inuit employees had been kept on staff to do maintenance work. With the money earned during construction days, many had bought boats, snowmobiles, motor sleds, and rifles; with equipment so much better than before, few saw any reason to give up hunting.

Otto had a good record of the health and nutrition of Cumberland Sound residents in the 1950s and wanted to find out the effect of wage employment. It was encouraging to find most people still in a good state of health.

Why had they escaped the "diseases of civilization"? There were good reasons to expect otherwise, as contact with outsiders had been going on before the arrival of Franz Boas in 1883. The first permanent whaling station had been established in the 1850s by William Penny at Kekerten Island on the north shore of Cumberland Sound. Infectious diseases introduced by whalers had decimated the population of Cumberland Sound, with less than 350 Inuit survivors by 1857 (Vlessides, 1997:301). But Otto believed that the people of Cumberland Sound, along with those from Holman Island, had been able to retain their social structure, as well as nutritional resources—traditional elements that were seriously eroded in the more urbanized centres of Iqaluit and Coppermine.

Otto found astounding differences in health among the four population groups in his study, apparently depending on the rapidity and the extent of the impact of Western civilization. Although they had the same genetic background, the people of Coppermine suffered from serious forms of TB three times more per capita than did those of Holman Island, where the traditional lifestyle still prevailed. Similarly, there was a far higher incidence of chronic ear infection and bad teeth in Coppermine people. Otto attributed these differences to diet.

Iqaluit fared the worst of any location with respect to the health parameters Otto measured. The only case of rickets that he encountered was also in Iqaluit, in a child whose parents were heavy drinkers. Sadly, it was one of many examples showing the detrimental effect of alcohol on the nutrition, as well as the physical and mental health, of children. As he had anticipated, Iqaluit had by far the lowest consumption of meat, the traditional Inuit food.

The conclusion seemed inescapable. Those people eating the traditional diet of game and fish got all the protein they needed and most of the calories, with little fat. They thrived. In strong contrast, those who consumed chocolate bars, potato chips, soft drinks, and high-calorie, low-protein starchy foods from the stores, were paying a heavy price. The most visible sign of deteriorating health was tooth decay, rampant in urbanized Iqaluit.

What bothered Otto as much as anything was the increased consumption of refined carbohydrates or sugars throughout much of the Arctic. People in one particular area under study were eating four times as much sugar as they had eight years before. Otto wrote about this in the magazine *Nutrition Today*:

> *The trend to the increased consumption of sugar developed over a century in Western nations; the shift has occurred, however, with almost a jolting abruptness in the last twenty years for the Canadian Eskimo.* (Schaefer, 1971:11)

Did this mean that Otto's Inuit friends in Coppermine and Iqaluit—and many other places for that matter—risked falling prey to the "diseases of civilization," such as heart disease, hardening of the arteries, obesity,

Nutrition and Malnutrition • 167

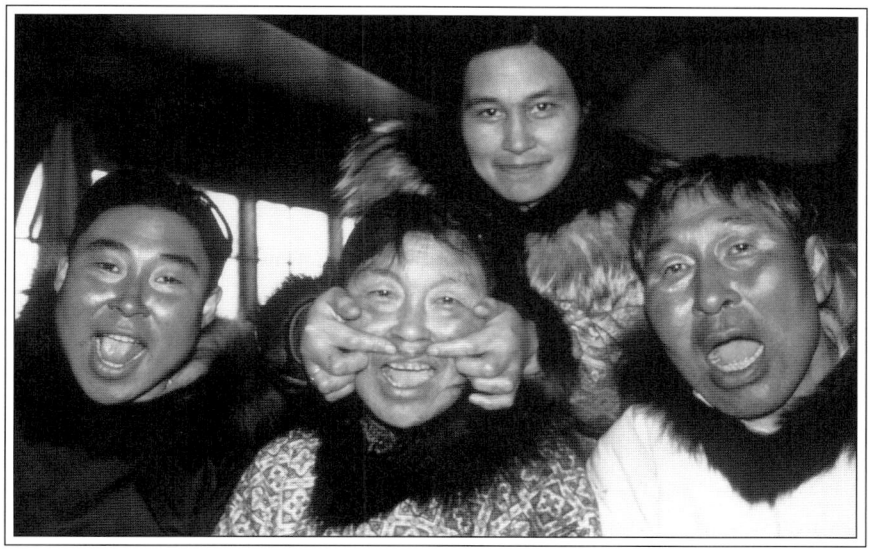

A family group from Walker Bay, north of Holman Island, photographed by Otto Schaefer in April 1965 to show their healthy teeth.

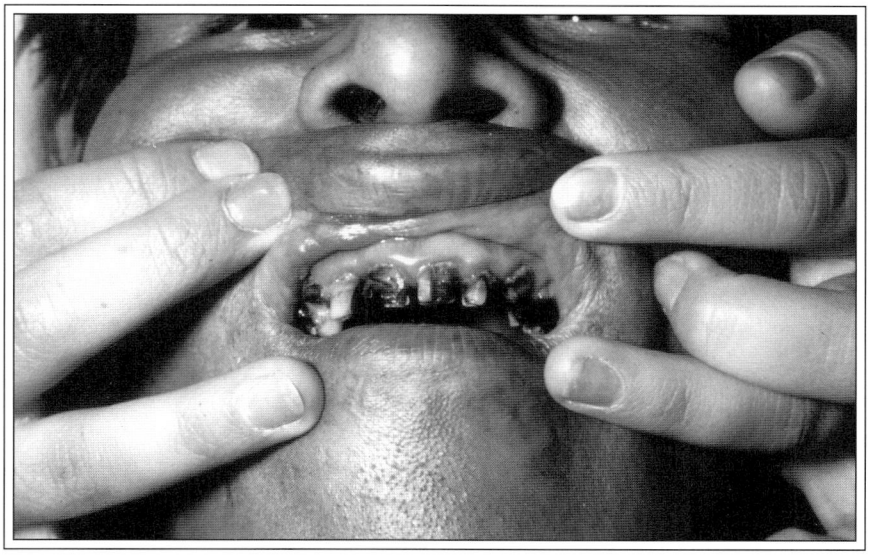

Badly decayed teeth of a resident of Iqaluit.

gall bladder disease, and diabetes? Enough evidence had accumulated to arouse his suspicions. His own research had found more cases of diabetes in one Mackenzie Delta area group than had been reported among all the Canadian Inuit a few years before. Further, he had seen x-rays of the legs of men over 40 who lived in the larger centres. Visible hardening of the arteries (calcification) occurred five times more often among these men than in men living in remote nomadic groups (Schaefer, 1971:14).

Otto believed that enticement to the Western diet and lifestyle exacted a heavy price: vulnerability to Western diseases. In addition, the new eating habits had pushed many Native people to the brink of malnutrition. Children and women of childbearing age suffered the most. "Education is the only solution to the problem, which at times approaches a level of self-inflicted genocide," he said (*Yukon News,* June 4, 1975:19).

33
A Changing and Crumbling Society

OTTO Schaefer grieved to see what was happening to the world of the Inuit, but he could not deny that there was some cause for rejoicing. The virulent epidemics of measles and smallpox of bygone years had ceased. Tuberculosis, the lingering, wasting disease that had kept the death rate higher than the birth rate for years, was rapidly knuckling under. When hunters came home empty-handed, few (if any) died from starvation: they simply bought food from the store. By 1973, Otto could write: "The gap between death and birth rates has been closed; the Inuit and Indians are no longer a disappearing people, but rather the fastest growing ethnic group in North America" (Schaefer, 1973:197).

Wonderful progress had been made. An untold number of lives had been saved, but at a staggering cost. Tuberculosis and famine were no longer the number one public health problems; alcohol abuse and venereal disease had taken over. Otto's initial suspicions were confirmed. Wherever the Inuit had moved out of sealskin tents and igloos into nice, oil-heated frame houses in locations where they fell so easily into the white man's ways, they had also fallen prey to the "diseases of civilization."

In Inuvik (an urbanized centre in the Western Arctic) for example, Otto measured the fat on young men, using calipers to take skin-fold measurements. He found a distressing number of overweight young men, three times the number per capita of distant Arctic Bay, where people lived the traditional way (Schaefer et al., 1980b). High blood pressure, almost nonexistent in Arctic Bay, threatened the health of several men and women in Inuvik. Similarly, tooth decay was widespread.

Gall bladder disease was approaching the incidence found in southern centres.

Bottle-feeding had become fashionable in places like Inuvik, but babies suffered for it. Otto had found a higher incidence of diarrhoea, chest infections, and ear infections in bottle-fed babies than in those still breast-feeding.

Increased sugar in their diet brought surprising changes in the growth of Inuit children. Otto found that growth acceleration during childhood produced adolescents that were two to four inches taller than the previous average for that age group. This was definitely not a sign of better health, he said, because the children were now getting very little protein in their diet.

Alcoholism continued to destroy the lives of its victims. "Forty percent of native men and women in Inuvik had a history of alcoholism leading to serious physical, legal or social consequences," wrote Otto in the *Canadian Journal of Public Health* (Schaefer et al., 1980b:397). Otto considered the surge in venereal disease to be mostly alcohol-related. At the same time, he recorded a dramatic increase in pregnancies among unmarried women, primarily teenage girls. Such pregnancies accounted for almost 50 percent of all births in the Mackenzie Delta.

"Eskimos Big Cancer Risk," read a 1975 headline in the *Edmonton Journal*. Otto was quoted as saying that their acceptance of the North American lifestyle might be the cause. "Lung cancer claims twice as many Eskimo men and 13 times as many women as in other Canadians," he said. He blamed heavy smoking superimposed on the common lung infections.

If abrupt acculturation was undermining the health of the Inuit, the assault on their social structure was even more deplorable. In the past, the individual person in the family was totally responsive to the needs of the family group in all his or her actions, even to decisions involving life and death. This meant complete interdependence, but with extreme personal tolerance.

Otto summarized the sad turn of events in a *Globe and Mail* article entitled "Modern Culture destroys Eskimo Family" (July 12, 1974). It was a gloomy report on Arctic life, and in the interview he held nothing back:

> *Once the proud hunter and provider, the father is now doing a menial job for the white man or worse still, he's surviving on handouts called welfare. Feeling useless and worthless, he resorts to drinking. Under the influence, he turns violent and often strikes his wife and children. Recovered, he feels remorse and [is] sometimes suicidal.*
>
> *The mother, once the indispensable centre of the family and always busy, buys her food and clothing in the store. With little to do, she idles away her time in movies, dances and bars.*
>
> *The infant, no longer breast-fed, lacks the intimate mother-child bonding and closeness. Later children get restless, confused by their parents …and unable to realize the desires awakened by school and movies.*
>
> *The family tends to drift apart, not needing each other so much. Irritability and anger are frequent. Children rebel against their elders.*

It was a hard indictment, but he had to say it. There was no denying that the basic elements of traditional Inuit society—a tightly knit family structure and personal values, attitudes, and practices shaped for successful life in a harsh environment—were falling apart.

The increasing number of suicides seemed to reflect the despair, despondency, and dislocation from the strong base the Inuit once knew. It was common knowledge that in the past many elderly people, feeling useless and unwilling to be a burden to their families, had walked out into a blizzard in the darkness or strangled themselves, sometimes with the help of an obedient relative.

Otto was well aware how Inuit felt the need to be "accepted" in their community, a heightened sensitivity to the judgement of others. One young man from Iqaluit had taken his life because others thought he had been careless in allowing his younger brother to fall from a cliff to his death.

At the trial for the murder of Soosee, Otto had learned of the suicide of her first husband, Josie. Josie had been charged with criminal negligence for not going to the aid of two women and three children whose igloo was buried by a massive snowdrift during a blizzard. Just the fact that he had been committed for trial was an indication that people suspected him to be guilty. In his mind he had been found "unacceptable." A few days before the scheduled court appearance, Josie left Soosee, walked out of their sealskin tent, and shot himself.

Dr. Gordon Butler, director of Health and Welfare's Northern Region, had drawn to Otto's attention the extremely high suicide rates among residents of the Northwest Territories, especially among the Inuit young people. Peaking in the 15–24 age group, the suicide rate for Inuit youth reached the tragic level of ten times that of non-Native young Canadians. Did this mini-epidemic of self-destruction indicate that the entire social fabric was ripping apart?

"We can't go back," said Guy Alikut, president of the Arviat Chamber of Commerce. "We would not want to go back. Our future is in taking charge of our land and our enterprises, and of making things work in a way that will benefit us, where we—not the government—make the decisions. And we may have to encourage our young people to move away if that is necessary for them to grow and develop" (Alikut, 1986).

Otto could see clearly his role—a very small one, he called it—to help redeem the people with whom he had so closely aligned himself. He would continue to study the ravages inflicted by Western civilization on their health and nutrition—and on their families and social structures—and to make his voice heard on their behalf.

If it meant a constant barrage of letters, newspaper and magazine pieces, articles in the medical journals, appearances before government officials, radio talks, and public presentations, then so be it. Otto would almost certainly find himself swimming against the tide. He might feel the sting of sharp criticism, as in the Yukon days when he battled to control alcohol abuse in Native people. But this was no time to give up.

34
Circumpolar Medical Conference

IN July 1974, hundreds of people from Scandinavia, the United States, the Soviet Union, and Canada—all countries with territory above the Arctic Circle—converged on the little town of Yellowknife (population 4500) for the Third International Symposium on Circumpolar Health. To take on the job of General Chairman, the Department of Health and Welfare chose Otto Schaefer. It would be his biggest task yet, and he wondered how he would cope with all the demands.

Previous conferences had been held in large university centres with fine facilities: the first at Anchorage, Alaska in 1968; the second in Oulu, Finland in 1971. Health professionals from many fields were invited to attend and present papers on health care in the Arctic setting. At Anchorage, Otto had presented what he called a "review paper" to the 80 or 90 delegates.

The initiative for the first conference had come from Dr. Earl Albrecht, then the assistant to the Commissioner of Alaska in charge of public health. Otto felt a remote kinship with Albrecht, a Canadian born in an Alberta town with a German name, Bruderheim. Believing that the vastly differing circumpolar countries shared common health problems, Dr. Albrecht could see the merit in an international meeting. It proved to be a valuable experience for all who attended.

At the second conference in Finland, Canada was asked to host the third conference, to be held in 1974. Some time later, Otto was officially requested to begin the planning and organizing. In spite of the obvious problem of logistics in a small, northern town—still a frontier town in many ways—he deliberately chose Yellowknife in the Northwest Territories. He wanted participation and active involvement of

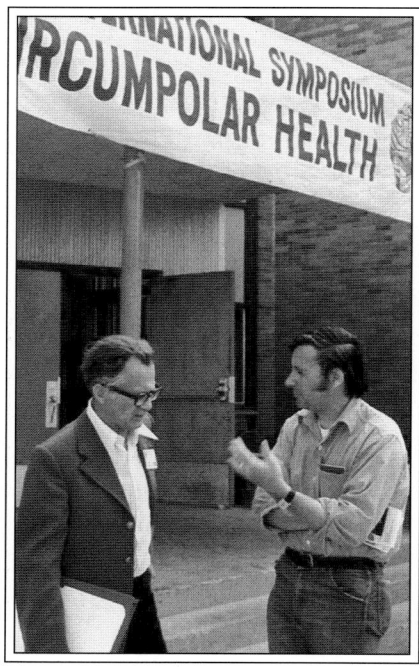

Dr. Otto Schaefer, Director of the Third International Symposium on Circumpolar Health, discussing matters with one of the delegates. Reprinted with permission from Nutrition Today 9(6), page 13, 1974.

Northerners, including aboriginals, working in health care. He hoped to get nurses and community health workers to learn all they could and to ask and answer questions.

Having worked closely with Dr. Jack Hildes on many projects, Otto considered him the ideal partner to help with this major undertaking. He asked Hildes to contact all delegates to the previous meetings, invite people to present papers, and supervise the overall scientific program.

Otto's most daunting task was to find suitable meeting rooms and accommodation for all the delegates. At that time, Yellowknife had only two small hotels and one ramshackle motel. He would have to make do with church basements and schoolrooms. Asking local citizens to offer bed and breakfast to foreign visitors would really put the legendary northern hospitality to the test.

Fortunately a government grant covered some of the costs, including the salary of a University of Alberta student who came to help as general manager. Mr. Stuart M. Hodgson, Commissioner for the Northwest Territories, provided much help and even arranged to have lapel pins made bearing the flags of all the countries represented.

Registrants began pouring in, altogether over 450 of them from all the circumpolar countries. The gracious people of Yellowknife opened their doors to welcome them.

But things got off to a shaky start at the opening Monday morning plenary session. Someone had forgotten to install the promised microphones and public address system. Otto had to race to the local radio station and borrow equipment.

In making arrangements for simultaneous translation into French and Russian, the sound technicians had provided cubicles for the interpreters and earphones for all the delegates. The technical part worked fine, but a political crisis threatened the whole operation. When the Soviet delegates learned that the Canadian government-appointed translator was the daughter of an anti-Bolshevik general, they grumbled *Nyet* and stomped off. Not until the committee wired for an official Russian translator from the United Nations in New York would they return.

With that small problem out of the way, the conference got into high gear and kept its momentum for all of the five days. The informal, small-town setting helped to relieve the stiffness of some medical meetings and delegates loosened their ties and mingled freely. Hildes and his committee had selected over 170 papers for presentation, many of high quality.

Some health problems existed in several countries, but there were also great differences. For example, while TB raged through the Canadian North in the 1950s, Saami from northern Sweden had remained free of the disease. And although all countries reported suffering from alcoholism, suicide and venereal disease, many Native people in Siberia (where 10 percent of the population were aboriginals) had refused to allow alcohol to be sold in their district. A speaker from Greenland commented that the rifle and snowmobile had made hunting easier, perhaps much too easy: game reserves were being depleted, threatening food supplies.

Some speakers stressed the value of involving more Native people in health care. In an initiative bearing some resemblance to the USSR's *Feldscher* program, young Inuit in the Canadian Arctic were being trained as community health workers. Returning to their community, they gave TB medication, taught public health principles, and served as liaison between the nurse-practitioner and the community. As if to illustrate the point, two Native community health workers and two nurse's aides presented papers relating their experience. Intimidated before the large international audience, they were quickly put at ease with a few encouraging remarks by the session chairman.

Otto did more than oversee the running of the conference. He submitted three papers of his own and another seven he had co-authored, including one with Father M. Metayer, author of several books on traditions and mythology of Central Arctic Inuit. Entitled "Eskimo Personality and Society: Yesterday and Today," that paper told the sad story of the erosion of family life (Schaefer and Metayer, 1976).

One of the undoubted highlights was the keynote address by 34-year-old Bill Mussell, a full-blooded Indian of the Skilak tribe (Mussell, 1976:3). Otto had met Bill in Ottawa at a conference called by Jean Chrétien, then Minister of Indian Affairs and Northern Development. Impressed by the young aide to the minister, Otto determined to invite him to Yellowknife as the theme speaker.

Bill Mussell gave a polished address to the large audience from many countries, and spoke from his heart, unafraid to "tell it like it is." He told of the need for mutual respect if anything worthy was to be accomplished for Native people. He approved heartily the training of Indian and Inuit people to meet their health needs, but it bothered him that the conference seemed to focus so much on problems. "I would like to see a conference held on positive things. What qualities do the Native people have? What strengths are there within their community?" he asked. Bill Mussell clearly made his mark among all the listening health professionals. They gave him a resounding standing ovation.

On Friday the conference concluded with a banquet that featured the celebrated drum dancers from the Mackenzie Delta and Dogrib Indian dancers from Fort Rae. After Otto's closing remarks, he too received a standing ovation from the assembly. While thanking the delegates for honouring him in this way, he was quick to acknowledge that the cooperation of a wonderful team accounted for his success.

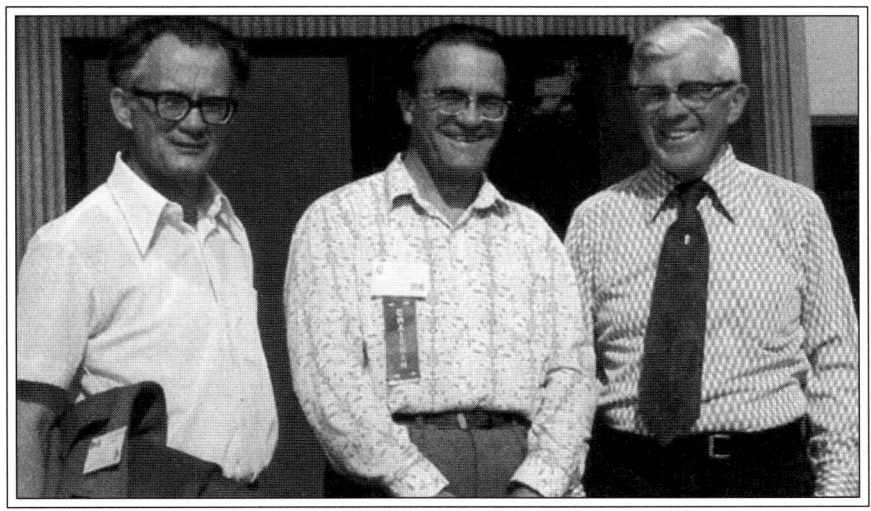

Otto Schaefer with Vlail Kaznacheyev from Novosibirsk, Russia and C. Earl Albrecht, M.D., who organized the First International Symposium on Circumpolar Health, held in Fairbanks in 1968. Reprinted with permission from Nutrition Today *9(6), page 13, 1974.*

When the proceedings of the conference were published, the editors gave Otto the credit for "carrying the heavy burden of initiating and supervising the progress of the symposium through to its successful conclusion" (Shephard and Itoh, 1976:xvii).

But for Otto, just as meaningful as the successful conference were the meetings with friends, old and new. Professor and Mrs. Henrik Forsius of Oulu University in Finland had become dear friends since the second conference, held in their city. Strangely enough, the Russian who had complained so loudly about the interpreter also became a good friend. Vladimir Ilyich Lenin Kaznacheyev ("Vlail" for short) was director of the Academy of Science in the University of Novosibirsk, Siberia. A tall, jovial, handsome fellow with a lively wit, he had once been an opera singer. But in the 1943 Battle of Stalingrad, when he was only 19, a serious head wound had shattered part of his skull. Military surgeons put in a silver plate to cover the big defect and told him he should never sing again, as the strain of reaching the high notes might damage his brain. He was also cautioned not to drink alcohol. As a doctor himself, however, Kaznacheyev thought he knew best. Back in Edmonton after the Yellowknife conference, he was one of several guests at Otto's home. After one or two glasses of wine, Kaznacheyev sat at the piano, leaned back, and burst into song. The chatter immediately ceased as his rich, warm baritone voice filled the whole room with an aria from *La Traviata*.

Kaznacheyev's main interests concerned human adaptation to the environment. He was certainly good company and a good friend, but Otto thought some of his ideas just a bit bizarre. Other delegates from the USSR admitted they could not fathom some of his weird concepts. Invited to his luxurious home in Novosibirsk four years later, Otto received great hospitality, and learned something else about his ruggedly independent host. In the lobby of his home hung a huge portrait of Stalin, about six times life-size. "The era of Stalin has gone. Your own government has put him aside," Otto commented, staring up at the massive portrait. "It will never be gone," pronounced Kaznacheyev. "He was the saviour of Russia."

35
At the Heart of Controversy

OTTO was never afraid to take an unpopular stance. "He was absolutely unafraid of speaking for or against something and risking criticism," said his daughter Taoya. More than one medical colleague looked askance at him for supporting and belonging to the Canadian Physicians for the Prevention of Nuclear War (CPPNW). "He's fraternizing with Communists," they said.

As an unflagging proponent of breast feeding, especially for Inuit mothers, he again ran afoul of others in his profession. In his opinion, breast feeding had a greater influence on the life and health of infants than any other single factor. He had not always thought so: in fact, in his early days at Aklavik, he spoke in favour of "a good and hygienically prepared formula." In time, however, he realized he was quite wrong; thereafter, he could not keep quiet. From his studies and surveys of health and nutrition in infants from many Arctic centres, he had ample evidence to support his views (Schaefer, 1974). And he considered it tragic that so many women readily adopted bottles and formulas "because it must be good if the white people are doing it."

Whereas babies suckling in the traditional way seemed to thrive, those on the bottle fell prey to one complication after another. Not able to get antibodies from their mothers' milk, these babies suffered far more often from chest infections and chronic discharging ears. Diarrhea was often a dangerous threat to health. In addition, anaemia occurred ten times more commonly than in breast-fed infants, a finding Otto reported at an International Congress of Nutrition in Prague in 1969 (Conway and Schaefer, 1969). Further, as a sign of their better nutrition, breast-fed infants walked on the average almost three months earlier than bottle-fed infants.

Otto saw another important reason for giving up the fashionable bottle feeding and going back to the traditional Inuit custom of breast feeding up until the age of three. This practice provided an effective type of birth control: the natural contraceptive action of lactation allowed for a desirable "spacing" of children. Some of his colleagues disagreed, saying, among other things, that such infants have difficulty accepting solid foods. They claimed their views were in line with prevailing medical opinion.

Otto replied that in all his years in the North, he had regularly seen mothers feed their infants finely cut meat and fish morsels, starting at eight months when breast milk tends to become inadequate. At one year, as appetite increases, they "eagerly munch the meat pulp," he wrote. He compared such robust babies with the "pale and pasty infants on nothing but bottle milk" (Schaefer, 1969).

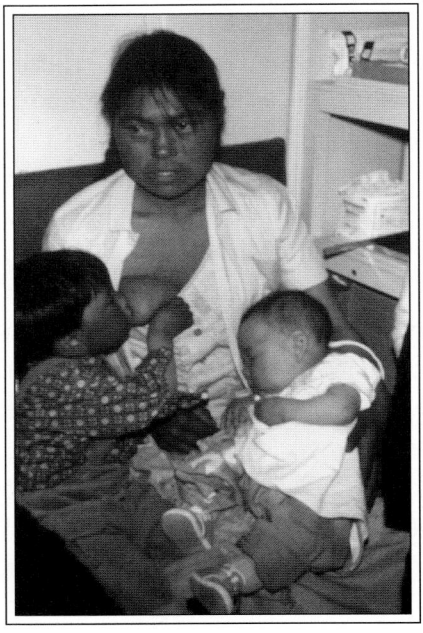

A Cape Dorset mother, after breast-feeding her youngest son, feeding her three-year-old son, on board the C.D. Howe *in July 1964.*

When he mentioned at a medical meeting that he had seen many mothers give their six-month-old children premasticated food, some voiced astonishment. "Surely it's not hygienic when the mother spits food into the baby's mouth," they said. Otto replied that the germs in her mouth would almost certainly reach the baby in any case. Besides, he added, immunity to those germs is probably transferred to the baby in the mother's milk.

He caused a much greater controversy, however, when he opposed the giving of iron to bottle-fed babies suffering from anaemia. A paediatric consultant from McGill University in Montreal had issued a policy that all babies in Baffin Island should be given "supplemental iron." At that time, the Faculty of Medicine at McGill oversaw the health care for Natives in the Eastern Arctic.

The supplemental iron program was an aggressive one, designed to correct the low blood haemoglobin that had become such a widespread problem. Undoubtedly it was well intentioned, but it caused an epidemic of diarrhea, a serious health hazard for infants. Looking back at the problem some years later, Otto was still fuming. "This professor had the worst influence you can imagine in the Arctic. She should have known that, in infants, iron encourages the growth of pathological organisms in the bowel that cause diarrhea," he said.

Otto sent a detailed memorandum (Schaefer, 1975b) to the head of the Department of Pediatrics at McGill and copies to all the doctors and nurses serving in the Eastern Arctic. The paediatric consultant phoned Dr. Butler, Regional Director for Health and Welfare, and snapped, "We don't want Schaefer interfering. Keep him away from Baffin Island."

McGill University had asked Dr. Butler for $200,000 to spend on research to find the answer to the widespread problem. It was Otto's turn to call Dr. Butler. "Just stop the iron and I think the problem will be solved," he said. Dr. Butler gave his approval, agreeing to assess the situation after two months. During that time, no cases were reported, and for the next year, they occurred only sporadically. The iatrogenic (doctor-caused) epidemic was over.

36
Native Women's Conference

IN 1981, a special event brightened Otto's life: an invitation to address a conference of Native women gave him a chance to return to his beloved Pangnirtung. The initiative came entirely from the women themselves. The Department of Indian and Northern Affairs contributed funding, but the women shouldered all the planning and organizing. And they came to Pangnirtung from far-flung places in the Western Arctic, Keewatin District, and Arctic Quebec. One of the prime movers was Bertha Allen from Inuvik. A housewife, she was born in Old Crow of Loucheux Indian parents and had married an Inuk. Otto remembers her as a person to be reckoned with.

Otto was not surprised that the women had planned the meeting. "They are more motivated and more willing than men to take bold initiatives," he said, "and they certainly seem much more anxious to do what is necessary to upgrade the quality of life in their own communities." The desire came not only from those with some schooling, but also from those with little or none. Well known by many of the women through his writings, lectures, and radio talks and his work in most of the Arctic centres, Otto was one of a handful of guest speakers asked to participate. But the planners had their own agenda and made it clear what topics they would like him to address. It turned out that they were interested in the same medical and social problems that Otto had been wrestling with. Many complained about having "too many kids around," one of the consequences of giving up breast feeding. Others found that they had little to keep them busy and that their children weren't respectful or obedient any more.

At the conference, the women spent much of their time in small discussion groups where they felt unafraid to talk freely about their lives. A group leader would report back to the gathered assembly afterward. Sometimes the sessions went on for hours, but everyone found out when they got too long. The honorary president was Attuat, a venerable Inuit matriarch from Arctic Bay, who was getting on in years. If a session was prolonged beyond her tolerance, she would fall asleep and snore like an elephant.

Several Native female community health workers who attended the conference spoke about their work and the changes they hoped to bring about. They welcomed the chance they had been given to assist the professionals and to provide the important liaison with the local community.

Otto addressed the conference on the subjects he knew best: nutrition and health, breast feeding, the threat to the family and society, and the problem of alcohol abuse. The latter happened to be the women's number one problem. "Drinking is destroying our family life," they lamented. Some admitted that they too had succumbed to the bottle to get away from feelings of uselessness and boredom. They all had stories to tell, many of them bitterly tragic.

One told the story of an Inuit wife who decided to solve the problem herself, with disastrous results. Ekootak, one of the best carvers and printmakers in Holman Island, had become addicted to booze. With money earned from his art work, he had ordered several bottles of liquor to be brought in by plane. But his infuriated wife got to the shipment before Ekootak, and smashed all

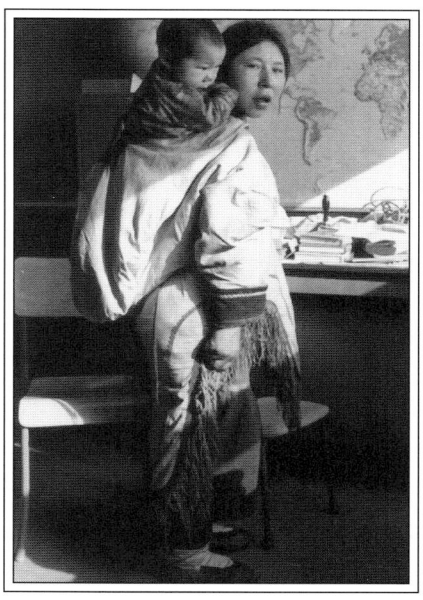

An Inuit mother attending school at Pelly Bay with her toddler in her amauti.

the bottles with an axe. That was too much for Ekootak, and he took his own life.

Otto told them about Itlaut, an exceptionally gifted man who figured in the book and film *The Land of Long Day*, shot on Bylot Island and produced in 1951 by the National Film Board of Canada. Originally Itlaut had worked as guide for Canon John Turner during his travels north of Spence Bay. Later the Department of Northern Affairs brought him down to a training centre in Alberta to teach outdoor survival in the cold. But it was at the Namao Air Force base near Edmonton, where he was instructing, that he started to drink in the officers' mess. Often he would come drunk to the Camsell Hospital, where his wife was a tuberculosis patient.

Otto took Itlaut to his own home in Edmonton a couple of times, trying to be his friend but also laying down the law. Itlaut tried to escape the habit, but he seemed doomed. Otto's last news about Itlaut came from Resolute Bay in the High Arctic, where he had settled. He had driven his snowmobile at high speed into a deep gully. Some time later he was found, bent lifeless over the steering column, with a fractured skull.

The curse of alcoholism seemed to rumble on like a juggernaut, dragging along to their ruin some of the finest members of Inuit society. Since his Whitehorse days, Otto had taken up arms—often in solitude—against the menace that found so many Northerners such easy prey.

But there were hopeful signs. The 1981 Women's Conference at Pangnirtung brought many hurting mothers, wives, and daughters into the battle. And some of them had success stories to tell: how they had managed to reduce or stop the drinking and violence of their husbands and sons—and themselves. They reminded everyone that women have always been the vital centre of all well-functioning Native families.

37
Didi

"WITHOUT her, Dad would never have had such a great career." So spoke Taoya of her remarkable mother, Editha or Didi. A polished and well-educated young woman, Didi had given up her urban environment and her own career in medicine to join her husband. She embraced the Arctic despite its hardships. Perhaps Pangnirtung was the place closest to her heart.

Didi's knowledge of Pangnirtung once averted a possible disaster. She was a passenger on a plane flying there from Iqaluit, when she saw that the pilot, new to the area, had no idea how to approach the narrow landing strip. He was worried about the strong downdrafts sweeping down from the mountains through the narrow fjord. Judge John Sissons, also a nervous passenger in the small plane, later wrote: "Our lady navigator knew the fjord well and guided us in to a safe landing" (Sissons, 1968:190).

From her youth, Didi had loved being outdoors. She and Otto had marvellous times in the Yukon skiing, hiking, and camping. "She always knew how to appreciate life with such vitality," her daughter Monika said of her.

"Otto had so many ideas swimming around in his head that he needed Didi to keep him from taking off," said Iris Stout, who worked with them in Whitehorse. Didi was the anchor Otto needed, and he depended upon her. Elva Taylor, Director of Nursing at the Camsell, remembers Didi gently chiding him: "Otto, you never remember where anything is!" or, "Don't forget to take such-and-such with you."

But later Didi was often alone with her young children while Otto toured on Arctic surveys anywhere between Holman Island and Arviat, or was far away presenting papers at conferences in Prague or Anchorage.

She never complained, and when others would say how much she had been sacrificing, she would accuse them of talking nonsense.

Didi was the centre of the family, the dynamic, loving mother who kept everyone together, whether her husband was home or not. Even when Otto was around, he seemed preoccupied with work. On picnics he would often sit in the car reading medical journals while the others were having fun. And in some ways, the family seemed happier when he was away.

"None of us felt close to our Dad when we were teenagers," volunteered one of the family in later years. Another said, "He used to get so short-tempered with us." Sometimes the children even considered leaving home and might have done so, had it not been for their mother. The girls suffered the most for "never doing anything right," but the boys also received little encouragement from their father. He would never say, "Well done, that's great!"

The family had to wait until company was present before they learned anything about the medical work that so absorbed him. When Otto made it clear that he would like Lothar to become a doctor, his son stoutly resisted. "I'll be anything but that," he said. He changed his mind only after spending holiday time in Germany with his maternal grandfather, a much-liked and respected family doctor.

The same man who was so widely honoured and admired—and loved—for his outstanding work on behalf of the people of the Arctic was, in the minds of his adolescent children, a failure as a father. Looking back on those years, Otto freely admits he did many things wrong. "If I had to do it again," he said, "I would have been a better family man. Now I can understand why Didi used to get so mad at me at supper time. I'd come home just in time, sit down at the table, and switch on the radio to get the news. Why didn't I have the sense to find out what the kids had done that day?"

Otto Schaefer was probably no worse a parent than many professional men whose families take a back seat. He was fortunate to have a jewel of a wife determined to see that her family got all the love, support, and encouragement she could offer. Happily, as the children grew older, father and family became reconciled. Friendship and happy relationships were permanently restored. And the whole family got together to plan and celebrate his 75th birthday in 1994.

In the summer of 1984, Otto and Didi made a return visit to Pangnirtung, something she had longed to do for 27 years. Many times she had talked about "our little white house surrounded at high tide on three sides by the breathing, heaving sea—the embodiment of paradise." It was to be a nostalgic farewell visit and would become for Didi a highlight of her life.

Flying up from Iqaluit, Otto had to explain to Didi that things would be different from 1957. During his 1965 and 1981 visits, he had seen how Pangnirtung had grown, how it had become an important centre for Inuit crafts, and how the hospital had closed down. And of course their little house had been moved away.

Otto had done his best to prepare her, but she still felt like a stranger in the town that had been her home. Yet somehow, a chill wind blowing off the bay made her feel that she had once belonged there. Even in July a stubborn fringe of tidal ice clung to the shore. The steep-walled fiord was ice-free, but snow and ice still whitened the jagged crags and pillars of the mountains beyond.

Paulusie, son-in-law of Etuangat, welcomed them to stay at his house, on a par with or even better than their lost white one. Etuangat, now 84, had lost some of his vision, but his eyes sparkled to see his old friend and partner, the man he had never considered his boss. He chuckled that since he was now the oldest resident, they should treat him with more respect. Nukinga, his senior by several years, had died many years before.

They hiked up the slope where Didi had broken her leg years before and gathered flowers that grew clustered deep in a gully. They went out in a boat, but this time not to hunt whales. They visited the centre where young men and women were carving beautiful soapstone and whalebone figures. They saw others weaving the now-celebrated tapestries, constantly in demand in the South.

The happiest times were socializing with old friends. They had taken along a projector and films from the early 1950s and invited everyone

188 • Sunrise Over Pangnirtung

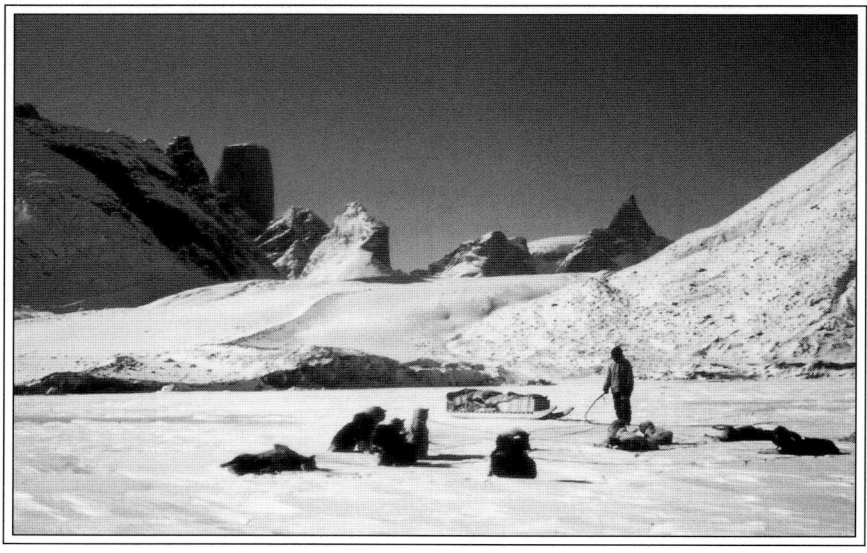

Etuangat and the dog team at Summit Lake in Auyuittuq National Park Reserve in spring 1957.

to come along to see what it was like in the old days. The schoolroom was packed to overflowing, and children outside peered through the windows, noses pressed flat. By popular request, Didi had to show the movies again the next night.

Then they embarked on the most strenuous backpacking hike they had ever done—climbing up the steep ravines above the fjord and mounting the hills to Auyuittuq National Park. Heavily laden with tent, sleeping bags, food, and extra clothing against the unpredictable weather, they found it hard climbing. They constantly had to cross streams and rivulets, surface meltwater that could not permeate the permafrost underneath. It took them six days to reach Summit Lake, where they pitched their tent on turf of soft moss. They cooked soup on a primus stove and also ate pilot biscuits and lean beef that Didi had dried herself. The next morning they awoke to find three inches of snow on the ground.

It was the wild, untamed wilderness that they both loved—craggy mountains, barren rocks and tundra, ice, and the ever-present chilling breeze. The glaciers of the Penny Ice Cap sparkled in the sun. They saw no terrestrial wildlife, but squadrons of seabirds wheeled and soared through the skies. They felt alone in the vast amphitheatre of mountains and rolling tundra. But for the whispers of rushing water, all was silent and still.

Suddenly the silence was broken by a strange and eerie sound, a human voice calling from afar. Dropping everything, they scampered over to the distant figure and found a man crawling on his hands and knees. Dirty and dishevelled, with sunken eyes and hollow cheeks, he wept to see them. He explained in French that his food had run out. He was famished and almost ready to give up.

Otto and Didi quickly shared some of their abundant food supplies with him. He explained that for days, his boots had been soaked from constant walking through bog and muskeg. It was impossible to walk in them. When he took them off, Otto could see that his feet were raw, blistered, and bleeding. He gave him bandages and the light sneakers that he kept to wear after a day of hiking. Slowly, they returned to Pangnirtung together.

Their new friend introduced himself as Dr. Wilfred Vitali, Head of the Department of Pediatrics at the Sorbonne in Paris. He had clearly learned a hard lesson from his misfortune in Auyuittuq National Park. Since that painful experience, this unusual man has travelled the length of the Mackenzie River valley down to the Beaufort Sea on foot, tracing the path of the great explorer. He has even trekked over most of the length of icy Ellesmere Island.

He told his two benefactors that he would never forget their gesture of kindness when he was in such desperate straits. True to his word, he has sent greetings and repeated expressions of gratitude every Christmas.

This trip proved to be Didi's farewell to her beloved Pangnirtung and the last time she would share backpacking with her husband. It could not have been a happier occasion, made all the more so with the knowledge that they had probably saved the life of an unusual but delightful professor of pediatrics from Paris.

38
Guest Lecturer

As Otto gained international stature as an authority on the health of the Inuit and their troubled society, he found himself constantly in demand as a speaker and lecturer. To return the hospitality shown to them in Yellowknife in 1974, the Russians invited him to be guest speaker at the next Circumpolar Conference, held in Novosibirsk, Siberia in 1978. Otto headed the Canadian delegation of twelve.

During the conference, Otto enjoyed good discussions with the Soviet Minister of Health, who had travelled from Moscow. They had met at the previous conference in Yellowknife. And the thorny Kaznacheyev, who had caused the translation crisis in Yellowknife, welcomed Otto as an old *drugi* (friend) and invited him out to his villa on the outskirts of Novosibirsk, a city the size of Montreal.

Some years later Otto received a special honour: he was selected to give the Knud Rasmussen Memorial Lecture in Copenhagen, Denmark before a large conference of authorities on health care in the polar regions (Schaefer, 1982b). In the Scandinavian countries and among circumpolar peoples generally, Knud Rasmussen was a heroic, almost legendary figure. Born in Greenland in 1879 of Danish and Inuit parents and educated at the University of Copenhagen, he spent 30 years of his life exploring the Arctic and studying the culture of the Inuit people. His principal interests were in demography (the statistical study of human populations), physical anthropology, and the study of cultural origins. In addition to trekking over much of Greenland, in 1923–24 Rasmussen travelled by dogsled across the mainland of northern Canada to Alaska and the Bering Strait, keeping a journal of meticulous travel notes. His Fifth Thule Expedition of 1921–24 resulted in the first detailed written account of the Inuit from the Keewatin District of the Central Arctic (Rasmussen, 1930).

Otto had a personal reason for accepting the invitation to give the Rasmussen Memorial Lecture. It was Rasmussen's *Groenlaendische Sagen* (Greenland Sagas) that had captured his fancy as a child. Rasmussen had done something else to command Otto's admiration. In 1923, during his travels by dog team across the northern wilds, he stopped while crossing Adelaide Peninsula, just south of King William Island. At the notorious Starvation Cove, where searchers had found bones and other relics of the men from the tragic Franklin Expedition, he paid tribute to these lost explorers. With the flags of Denmark and Britain flying at half-mast, he read the burial service for their remains, which had lain neglected for three-quarters of a century. "The whole world is the tomb of brave men," he said. Thus it seemed fitting that the bones of men of English, Scottish, and Irish descent should receive the dignity of last rites from a Greenlandic Dane (Neatby, 1958:186).

Otto began the Rasmussen Memorial Lecture by admitting that many in the audience "are much more worthy of this honour and are better qualified than I am to celebrate the memory of Rasmussen." He then went on to review Rasmussen's life, focusing on how much the explorer had learned by living with and listening to the Inuit. His goal was to link Rasmussen's work in demography with his own observations on the origin and effect of illnesses. Findings from Rasmussen's studies of Inuit populations in the early 1920s had helped to answer his own questions about current demographics.

Studying the 1961 Inuit census figures, Otto had wondered why women aged 30 to 44 years numbered 20–35 percent fewer than men of that age group. Could something have happened back in the 1920s or later that selectively affected girls? Rasmussen's studies gave him the answer: female infanticide. At that time, girl babies were simply left out in the snow, for reasons that the Inuit felt they could justify. With the advent of missions, trading posts, and police detachments, the practice came to an end.

But the 1971 census figures also showed the same disparity in the number of middle-aged women as compared to men. Could there have been some other factor that reduced the number of women? Again Otto found the answer—the old enemy, tuberculosis. While almost all Inuit in the Canadian Arctic were exposed to TB in the 1940s and 1950s, young women of child-bearing age were most vulnerable to the disease and most likely to die from it.

Another factor of somewhat lesser importance accounted for the smaller number of women. Otto had seen more than his share of women haemorrhaging severely after childbirth. He and Etuangat had raced their dogs across frozen Cumberland Sound to reach one such young woman. She had survived, but he wondered how many others had not been so fortunate.

When it came to comparing male:female ratios in the 60–65 age group, he found that not only had gender equality been achieved, but women were beginning to outnumber men. He attributed this to the repeated attacks of "frozen lung" that affected hunters, eventually causing their death around age 60.

Otto took the opportunity to bring before the audience a favourite theme: breast feeding. Rasmussen had described "the traditional small Inuit family of three-four children" in 1925, when all mothers nursed their babies. The alarming rise in birth rates started in 1955, when "development" brought cash income, baby bottles, and milk powder to the North. He concluded his address by once again acknowledging the groundbreaking work of Knud Rasmussen and expressing regret that the great explorer, ethnologist, and writer could not have lived longer. Rasmussen returned exhausted from his last expedition in 1933; he was only 54 when he died that fall.

39

Honoured by the North

ON Thursday, November 26, 1981 a crowd gathered in the building occupied by the Department of Health, Government of the Northwest Territories, in Yellowknife. The Dr. Otto Schaefer Health Resource Centre was to be officially opened. Guests included John Parker, Commissioner; Arnold McCallum, Minister of Health; and Dr. J.D. Martin, Regional Director of Medical Services. The special guest, of course, was Otto Schaefer, honoured for his "outstanding contributions to the health care of northern Native populations."

The official dedication and ribbon-cutting ceremony gave Otto little satisfaction, but he inwardly rejoiced that there was now a broad-based resource of books, journals, pamphlets and other materials for health care workers in the Arctic. His own contributions to the medical literature were included, as well as the proceedings from the various circumpolar conferences and papers written by Dr. Jack Hildes and other researchers.

Doctors and nurses from the Stanton Hospital in Yellowknife would have access to the Resource Centre, and nurse-practitioners from the remote stations could phone in and ask for materials. The Resource Centre officially declared itself available to help "health professionals, allied health groups, Native organizations, schools, and the general public."

Yellowknife's *News of the North* (November 26, 1981), which reported the event with a picture of Otto cutting the ribbon and a resumé of his career, referred to "the years when he was often the only doctor for many miles to treat several thousand residents." The article went on to say: "His research studies among northern native populations have earned him worldwide recognition as a leading authority in the health field."

Four years later, he returned with Didi to Yellowknife, to receive "The Commissioner's Award for Public Service at the Highest Level" at

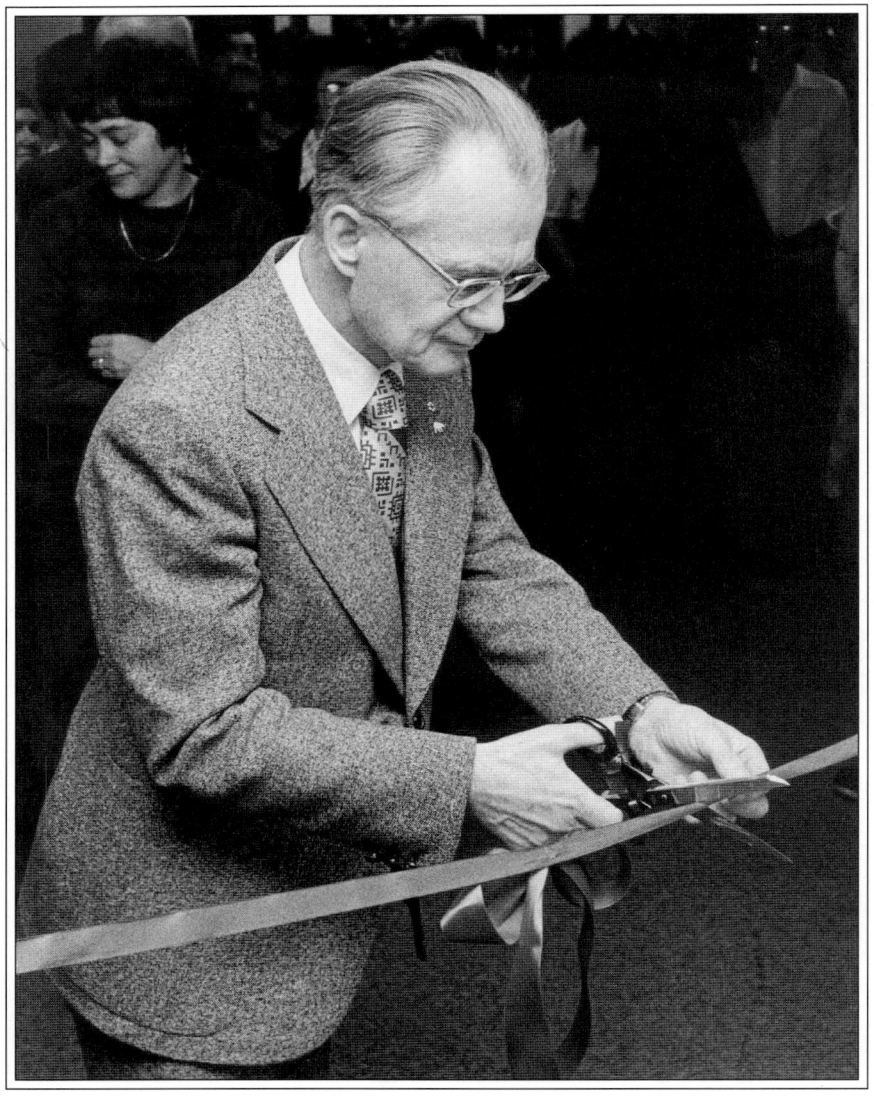

Otto Schaefer cutting the ribbon at the opening of the Dr. Otto Schaefer Health Resource Centre in Yellowknife. November 26, 1981.

a special ceremony (*Hay River Hub*, June 5, 1985). Guests invited to share in the celebrations included medical colleagues and nurses from the area as well as members of the Water Board of the Northwest Territories, on which he was serving. When told he could invite guests from Edmonton, Otto declined, wanting to avoid the expense. Didi, of course, had to be there. Her presence at his side, along with that of friends and colleagues, put this award near the top of his long list of honours. The celebration dinner, a relaxed and informal affair, included at Otto's request some tasty Native delicacies.

He also felt honoured to be sharing the occasion with the family of a young woman receiving posthumously the Commissioner's Award for Bravery. Denise Drybones of Fort Rae had died during the previous winter while trying to rescue her grandmother and two children from a burning house.

In making the presentation to Otto, Commissioner Parker commented that "few people today remember that when Dr. Schaefer practised medicine in the North, it was a different world, with airplanes once a month, radio messages by key, fresh food for only two months of the year, and a holiday 'outside' every two to seven years." Citing Otto's accomplishments, the commissioner presented to him a plaque that read:

The Commissioner's Award for Public Service at the Highest Level is presented to Otto Schaefer CM, MD, FRCP of Edmonton, Alberta in recognition of his outstanding contribution to improving the health and nutrition of northern residents through more than 30 years of dedicated and compassionate service. From his ministering to the sick at Pangnirtung and Aklavik in the early 1950s and more latterly through his research in medical work with the Northern Medical Research Unit, he has demonstrated continuing dedication and medical excellence in improving the health and well-being of northern residents.

   (Signed) John H. Parker,
Commissioner for Northwest Territories
May 23, 1985

40
Papers and Publications

"WHENEVER I came across something interesting, I pulled out my notebook." A constant companion right from the days of his youth, the notebook—with scribbles sometimes in English, sometimes in German—recorded not just Otto's widespread interests, but also his insatiable curiosity.

Actually, he had two notebooks. In one he recorded observations about the Inuit and the Arctic in general. The other he filled with information about patients, their illnesses, and their lifestyles. Often there were puzzling questions. Why did the health of active, vigorous hunters deteriorate after age 40? Why were children in the Central Arctic so susceptible to meningitis? Were there reasons for the high suicide rate? Had the Inuit always been so honest and trustworthy?

He wrote down some of the impressive Native practices, such as applying spruce gum to the terrible wounds of a bear mauling. It intrigued him that one elderly woman had learned how to remove pieces of retained placenta after childbirth and had undoubtedly saved the lives of many young mothers. Although the idea didn't appeal to him personally, he could see the wisdom of eating the stomach contents of slaughtered caribou to obtain scarce vegetable matter and vitamins.

Most of all, he noted the changes in eating habits, nutrition, and lifestyle since his early days in the North. Life was more comfortable and less hazardous; but why were so many young men getting paunchy, and why did they drink so much? Why were so many bottle-fed babies sickly and anaemic? What had happened to the once strong and wholesome Inuit family structure?

The end result of a lifetime of questioning, examining, travelling, and studying was astounding: more than 100 papers and monographs published in medical and paramedical journals, as well as contributions to books (see Appendix). Many of these publications were the result of original studies in the nutrition and general health of Native peoples. Others were concerned with infectious diseases, the effect on the lungs of exposure to cold, and changes in lifestyle and culture. He sought the collaboration of other workers involved in northern health care and research and co-authored some papers with them. It certainly was not "ivory tower" research with little practical application. He aimed to make his results and conclusions known by regularly informing personnel serving with the Government's Medical Services Branch and by personal involvement in educational programs in northern settlements.

His first article had opened the eyes of the North American and European medical world to health needs in the Canadian Arctic. His last, "The Changing Health Picture of Inuit and Indians in the Northwest Territories from the 1950s to the 1980s" (Schaefer, 1994), was no less worthy. A wide-ranging review of the tumultuous years with their good and not-so-good changes, it began with a personal comment on Otto's boyhood fascination with northern peoples after reading Franz Boas's *The Central Eskimo*. To drive home a point he had promoted relentlessly for years, he included a picture of two Inuit women from Pelly Bay, happily nursing their infants.

Otto had always considered Dr. Jack Hildes as the man to whom he owed the most for advice and help with his research and writing. Hildes had "torn apart" that first 1959 paper, citing shortcomings and deficiencies. They crossed swords again before realizing they were really kindred spirits.

Hildes's original training in physiology had spurred his interest in adaptation to extreme cold. Otto admired his knowledge, thoroughness, medical skills and habits of hard work, as well as his interest in and understanding of Native people, especially their social and medical problems. It was while they were both working aboard the *C.D. Howe* during the 1957 Eastern Arctic Patrol that Hildes explained to Otto his work on the subject of shivering. He had travelled to the Kalahari desert in South Africa to observe a group of Bushmen that usually slept half-naked. Otto told him how Etuangat's young son was given a thin, almost hairless piece of caribou hide to lie on at night—to train him to sleep in the cold, his father said.

It was Jack Hildes who encouraged Otto to go to the University Hospital, Edmonton to complete the training required in Canada for his specialty in internal medicine. When Otto's research work began in earnest in 1964, he received great encouragement and practical help from Hildes and his colleagues at the University of Manitoba.

The megaproject of their collaborative efforts was the Yellowknife Circumpolar Conference of 1974 that brought hundreds of delegates from the Soviet Union, the United States, Scandinavia, and Canada. Otto had served as general chairman, while Jack worked as chairman of the important scientific program.

From the beginning Hildes had taken a novel, almost radical, approach: he put forward the idea that Native communities should be involved in their own health problems and encouraged to discuss their health care priorities. He induced community members to voice their complaints and contribute to the formulation of new health care policies. And like Otto, he stressed "the superior value and special need to preserve breast feeding."

Schaefer and Hildes co-authored 26 papers on medical and social research among the Inuit without a serious disagreement. But their friendship and fruitful collaboration came to an end in 1984. Otto was the first to spot something wrong: he noticed that his usually indefatigable friend would suddenly turn bleary-eyed, fall asleep, and start to snore. He would re-awaken, only to repeat the deep drowsiness. In due course Hildes underwent surgery to remove a brain tumour. He recovered, but after living as a semi-invalid for several months, he died in 1984.

41
Full Circle

HE was reaching the time of life for turning the hunting over to the young men, as his Inuit friends would say. But Otto felt he was still good for a few more seals, or maybe the odd caribou.

In 1980 he was appointed to the Water Board of the Northwest Territories as medical consultant. The job didn't seem onerous, but it carried heavy responsibilities. The Board had to make important decisions concerning safe water supplies, waste disposal, and the impact of industrial development on the environment. The seven-person Board included an Indian, an Inuk, and representatives from the Department of Indian Affairs and industry. Frequent public hearings allowed the Board to hear all points of view. Often when it was a case of the Natives versus the industrial companies, decisions were hard to make. Indians and Inuit were tempted by the offer of jobs, but what if the new industry polluted the water and destroyed the fish?

The Berger Commission of 1977 faced a similar dilemma. To supply Beaufort Sea oil to large markets in the south, a consortium of companies had proposed an oil pipeline that would run along the Mackenzie River and the Alaska Highway. Asked by Justice Berger to submit a report, Otto expressed his concern not only for the environmental impact but also for the harm to the Native way of life. In the end, Berger recommended a 10-year moratorium on the project. In those ten years, world market conditions would change, making it too expensive to extract the Beaufort oil.

With advancing years, Otto's promotion of conservation and respect for the environment intensified. He and Didi deplored wastage of any kind and would throw things out only when they were hopelessly beyond recycling. "He would even inspect the compost to make sure that every apple had been eaten right down to the bare core," said Taoya. Otto also deplored pollution of any kind, including the raucous roar of the "abominable snowmobiles," as he called them. These noisy machines were a great asset for hunting caribou in the North, he wrote in a letter to the editor of the *Edmonton Journal*, but they had no place in the city of Edmonton.

The year set for Otto to retire from the Department of Health and Welfare was 1984, but he was asked to stay on for another year. Then he was told to plan a last trip to Ottawa, for a retirement dinner and a unique honour. Didi had been with him when he received a previous honour in Ottawa: the Order of Canada. At a ceremony in Government House on January 14, 1976, Governor General Jules Léger had pinned the medal of the Order on his chest. But when His Excellency attempted to shake his hand, Otto felt something "give." Lacking a dress suit, he had borrowed one from his neighbour, a man of somewhat broader girth. A safety pin had solved the problem, but it chose the moment of the handshake to spring open. Fortunately, a frantic snatching gesture with Otto's left hand saved the borrowed pants from hitting the floor.

The brief citation for the Order of Canada read: "A physician whose love of the North and its people has manifested itself in his service to the sick in the Northwest and Yukon Territories for many years." At home, the *Alberta Report* (January 26, 1976) noted the award under the headline "Honours for a Distinguished Edmontonian," and showed a picture of white-coated Otto, describing him as "a man desirous of a better country."

Dr. Maurice Beare, a former colleague of Otto's from Camsell days, recalls attending the "posh farewell retirement dinner" for Otto and Didi Schaefer on December 10, 1985. The Westin Hotel in Ottawa was full of dignitaries, including Dr. Lyell Black, from the Department of Health and Welfare, and The Honourable David Crombie, Minister for Northern Affairs. Vera Roberts was there, not as a dignitary, but as a special friend and colleague who had proved invaluable to Otto in the operating room at Pangnirtung 30 years before. Dr. Beare remembers that after the delightful dinner "several distinguished speakers stood up

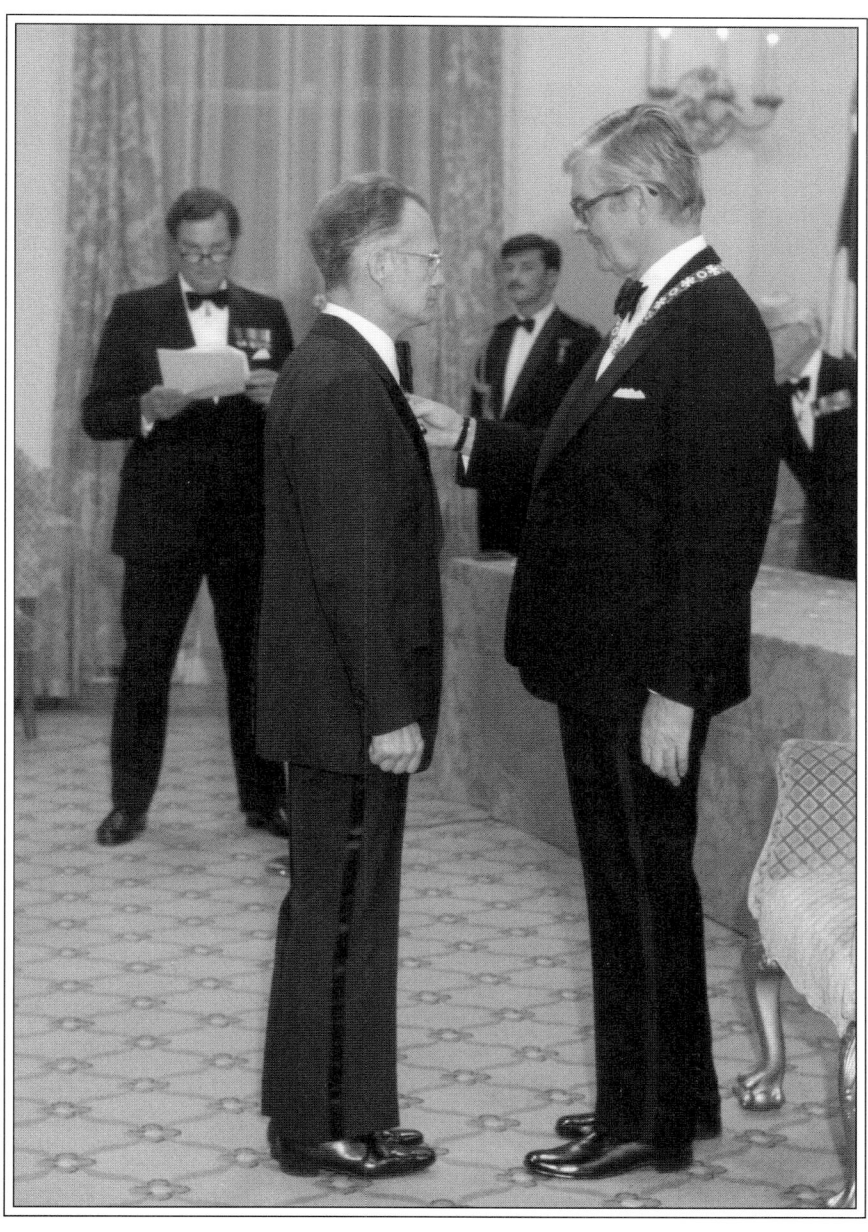

Otto receiving the Order of Canada from Governor General Jules Léger. Credit: John Evans Photography Ltd., Ottawa. #12300/134.

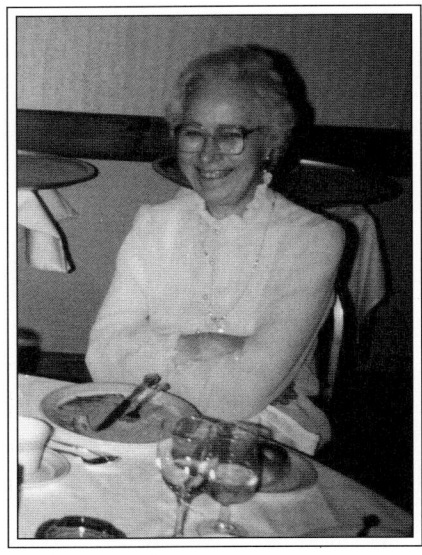

Vera Roberts at the farewell dinner for Otto, held in Ottawa in December 1985.

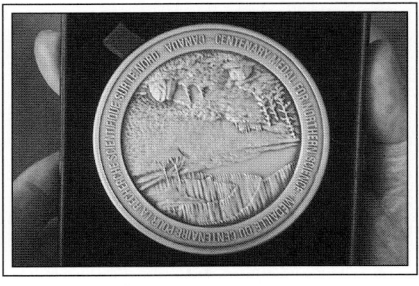

The Northern Science Award Centenary Medal. Photo by Gerald Hankins.

and praised the work of the man now retiring."

After offering expressions of gratitude as best he could, Otto tried "to bring things down to earth" and to give credit where he thought it really belonged.

Now is the time to tell you the old Inuktitut proverb, he said. "A hunter—or any man for that matter—can only be as good as his wife allows him to be. If your wife is a good seamstress and sews your fur clothing together well, you can run in it for long stretches, chasing your game until you catch it. But if she makes poor clothing, it will fall apart and you will freeze. So even in the Inuit society, where the hunter is so venerated, everyone realized that the housewife and mother was not only the centre of the family, but also the indispensable partner for the hunter."

During the evening set aside to honour Otto and Didi Schaefer, gifts were showered upon them, including a beautiful blanket woven in Pangnirtung. The highlight of the evening was saved for last, and for Otto and Didi it would be one of the most precious moments of their lives. The Honourable David Crombie presented Otto with the prestigious Northern Science Award and Centenary Medal and a cheque for $5000. Included in his ten-minute presentation address were the following comments:

> *Dr. Schaefer has dedicated his career to the study of health care for Native people in the North. I am pleased to honour him with this award in recognition of his outstanding contribution to medical science and health care in the North.* (Indian and Northern Affairs Canada, 1985)

Suddenly after all these years the name of Otto's boyhood hero, Franz Boas, was figuring in his life again. In September 1883, toward the end of the First International Polar Year, Germany had sent Boas to Baffin Island to map the little-known Cumberland Sound. Now Otto held in his hand a handsome medal commemorating the work of that first polar year. Boas's illustrious publications were major contributions to Arctic and Inuit studies. They also happened to set the course for the life of a young boy from Betzdorf, Germany.

42
Cruel Blows

OTTO and Didi loved all their children dearly, but their youngest—as is the case in many families—was special. At age 24, Heidi was the embodiment of so many fine Schaefer qualities, and more. She skied, canoed, kayaked, hiked, and climbed mountains—and did everything with zest. Her second home was the wilderness, and she was a committed member and volunteer with the Canadian Parks and Wilderness Society. When asked why she and her siblings were such rabid environmentalists, she answered without hesitation, "It's because of our parents."

Heidi loved life and took it seriously, displaying a maturity beyond her age. Trained as a physiotherapist, she could have afforded comforts and luxuries, but she chose the simple life and owned little besides a not-so-new truck.

Sadly, it was Heidi's love for the mountains that brought her sparkling life to an end one day in December 1988 (Dodge, 1989). She and a friend, Ken Wallator of Jasper, were climbing Mt. Balanger, a 3050 m peak in Jasper National Park. At a point only 120 m below the summit, they stopped on a ridge to rest and take a picture. When Heidi stepped back for the picture, a cornice of snow gave way and she plunged down the mountainside. Ken hurried down and tried to carry her through a snowstorm to a climbers' hut some distance below. But Heidi died in his arms as he staggered down the rocky slope towards the hut. Because darkness was closing in, he could not go for help until the next morning.

The first person in the family to get news of the tragedy was Heidi's sister Monika, who worked as a warden in Jasper National Park. Monika immediately called her parents in Edmonton. The bad news left Didi hanging her head and sobbing; Otto was so overcome that he slumped to the floor. It was devastating news, as anyone who has lost a child can testify.

Heidi left the sum of $3000 in her bank account. With a matching amount from her parents and contributions from others, the Heidi Schaefer Wilderness Preservation Award was established. Every year a cash award is presented to a Parks and Wilderness volunteer who has shown genuine commitment to conserving the environment.

The loss of exuberant and lovable Heidi was a cruel blow for both of her parents, but Didi was the first to come to terms with the loss and to accept it without bitterness. In a phone conversation with Elva Taylor she said, "We have to remember that she died a happy person in her beloved mountains, doing what she liked best of all. It was a blessing to have had her for 24 years." Not for a moment was Didi prepared to blame anybody or anything for her death.

The loss of Heidi came on top of another impending tragedy. Always a good hiker, Didi had shouldered her 35-pound pack with ease when she and Otto camped in rugged Auyuittuq National Park on Baffin Island for ten days in 1984. She certainly didn't lack energy, but soon afterward Otto noticed strange features in her appearance. She developed an abnormal fullness of

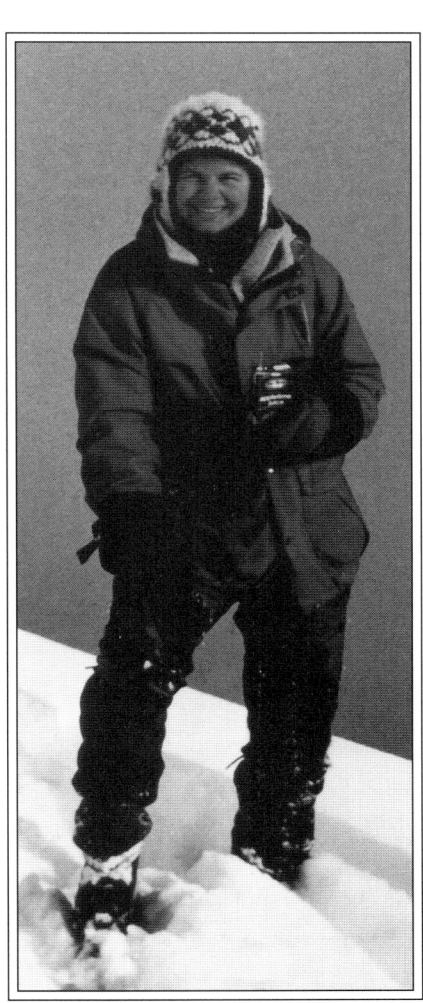

Heidi Schaefer.

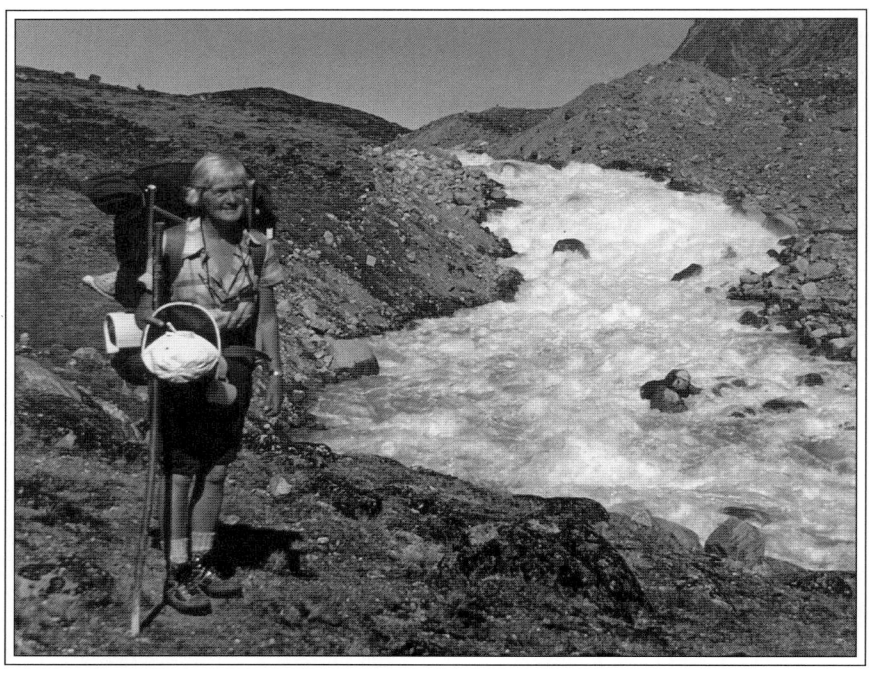

Didi Schaefer on July 21, 1984 during the Schaefers' walk to Summit Lake.

her face and a wispy beard of facial hair. A sort of hump appeared at the base of her neck. Later she developed symptoms of high blood pressure. What did these unusual features mean?

Otto took her to the University Hospital in Edmonton, where an endocrinologist diagnosed a tumour, possibly malignant, of the adrenal gland. The news shook them both. Facing surgery for a life-threatening disease, Didi told her old friend Betty Amerongen, "I mustn't die. Otto needs me." In 1985, Dr. Alan McCarten operated. He found and removed a "low-grade tumour of the adrenal gland," reported later by the pathologist to be noncancerous. Her life was not endangered.

Didi enjoyed good health for the next few years, but Heidi's death seemed to bring about a recurrence of her previous signs and symptoms. Dr. Tom Williams from the University Hospital performed a second operation and removed the tumour that had recurred. When more worrisome signs appeared a couple of years later, a chest x-ray showed that the tumour, once thought to be noncancerous, had spread to her lungs. The end could not be far away.

By 1989, Otto had given up most of his work commitments to care for his wife, who had been such a staunch supporter for 37 years. It was a complete reversal of their usual roles and weighed heavily upon him. She grew weaker but continued to look on the bright side and make the best of whatever each day offered. One day she said, "I may be dying of cancer, but I don't have any pain and my joints aren't stiff and arthritic."

She refused to give up her outdoor adventures, even if she couldn't carry a pack any more. In 1990, at age 62, she took a three-day canoe trip with her son Lothar and his wife, travelling downstream through the Mackenzie Delta from Inuvik to the Beaufort Sea. When her strength was fading, it was the outdoor adventures that sustained her, said Betty Amerongen.

On April 22, 1992, the day before she died, Didi climbed into a canoe at Devon for the trip down the North Saskatchewan river to Edmonton. Just gliding by beaver dams and hearing the honking of Canada geese overhead filled her heart with joy.

The *Edmonton Journal* of May 2, 1992 devoted a half page to this fine woman, whose life "brimmed with vitality." In the article, Monika spoke for all the family when she said of her mother: "Her sense of humour and positive attitude were always there…She was more than a mother to us: she was our friend…There was no generation gap with her."

Otto could not deny that her loss was the cruellest blow that life had ever dealt him. She had "always been there" and now she was gone. For a time all his achievements in the North, all his awards and honours, and all the expressions of acclaim and praise felt like cold, grey ashes. Numb and confused, he wandered around without direction. All the meaning had been sucked out of life.

He did eventually recover, but of course life was never quite the same again. As his colleague Dr. Edwards was to say, "He is a man of deep resources and great energy and still wanted to make the best of the years left to him."

43
Etuangat Elevated

[My father] respected the Inuit and tried his best to learn from them. He admired them especially for their ability to survive in the harshest climate and environment on earth. Few people he respected more than Etuangat.

Taoya White

IN November 1995, Etuangat made his first journey to the South, to Ottawa. There the white-haired, 95-year-old Inuit patriarch donned a bow tie and tuxedo to shake the hand of Governor General Roméo LeBlanc and receive the Order of Canada. The citation read:

He is a living link with the past, whose experience as a whaler and with the old ways of hunting and fishing has been invaluable to his people and to all who wish to understand the Inuit culture. His knowledge of weather, ocean, land and ice conditions and his skills in living on the land have helped the Inuit survive during a period of rapid and tumultuous change. (Office of the Governor General, 1995)

Senator Willie Adams, an Inuk from Arctic Quebec long settled in Rankin Inlet, took Etuangat on a tour of the Senate and the House of Commons and arranged for him to visit the Experimental Farm in Ottawa. There he saw his first horse and watched a calf being born. The owner promptly named the calf in his honour.

He saw his first tree, and then thousands more. But he wasn't overly impressed: "One tree by itself is very nice," he said through an interpreter. "But when they're all crowded together, they block the view."

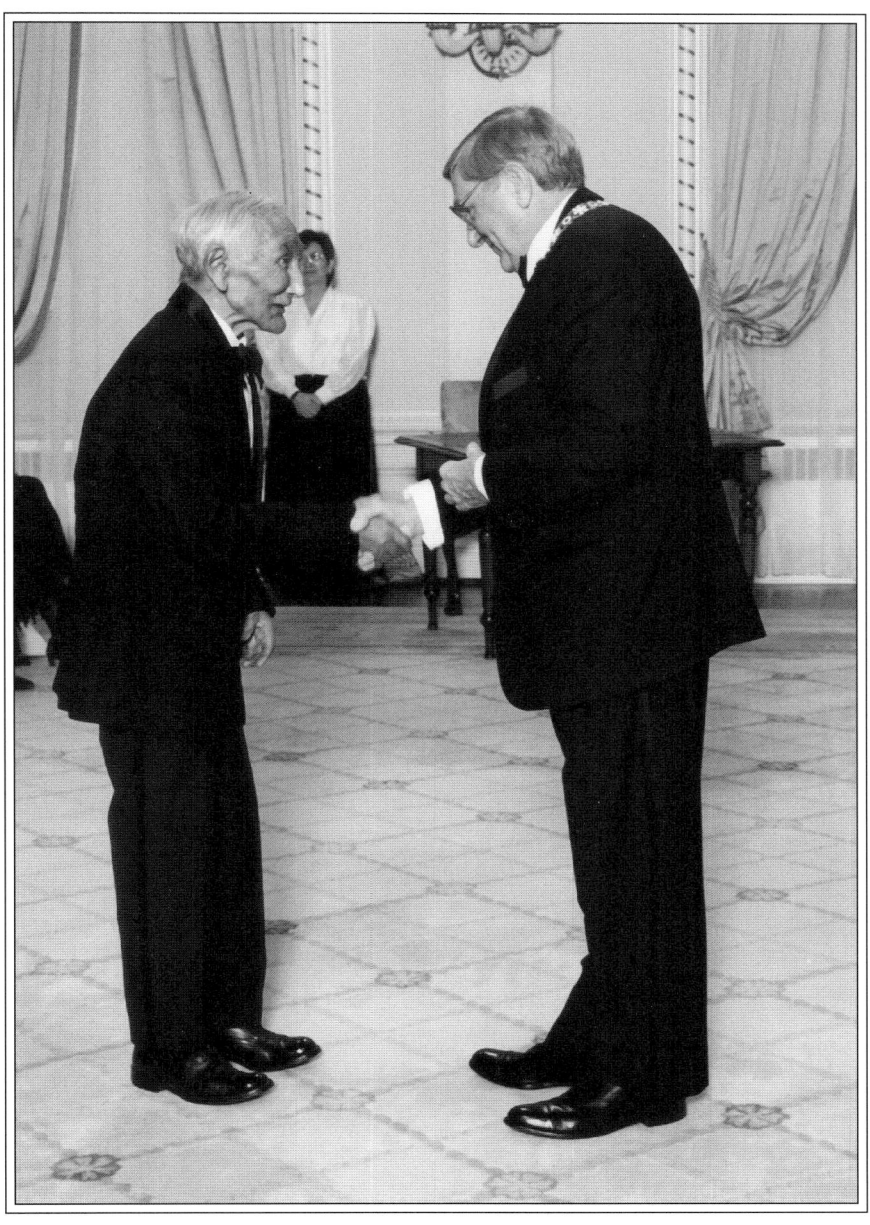

Etuangat receiving the Order of Canada from Governor General Roméo LeBlanc on November 16, 1995.

Some time later, the whole community of Pangnirtung gathered to honour Etuangat (*Nunatsiaq News*, January 5, 1996). As a reflection of the changing times, he wore a suit and tie for the occasion. Honoured as "one of the most respected elders in the Baffin region," he was described as being known all his life as a helper, traveller, and one of the best hunters of the last four generations.

Bright and alert, Etuangat told the gathering about the time he had travelled by dog team across the Cumberland Peninsula to get help for his sick wife. While they were there at Pangnirtung's mission hospital, he was offered a job. It was a tough job, they warned him. As a guide and helper, he would need to travel by dogsled from Pangnirtung to all the camps and settlements in the region. But he took it on, probably because "I loved to learn and participate."

For decades he worked and travelled as the doctor's helper, journeying over the mountains and across the fjords. During an epidemic in the

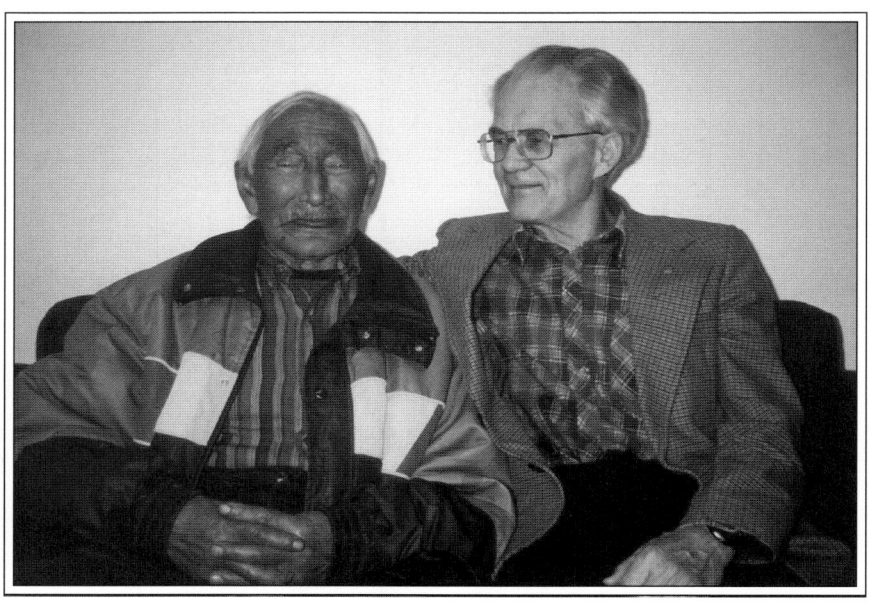

Otto Schaefer and Etuangat (aged 93) during Otto's last visit to Pangnirtung in 1993. Photo by Jane George.

1940s he worked for three days without sleep, helping to give inoculations and transporting the sick to hospital. "When you see so many sick people, you want to help in whatever way you can, and I did my best," he said. During all those years he never had a single accident or disaster. "I feel a bit proud of my success, because nature is so unpredictable," he said.

Etuangat concluded his talk to the community with some advice "to all the young people complaining about being bored": "Young people with nothing to do should make themselves busy...There is so much to learn, and it would build their confidence."

On January 16, 1996, Etuangat died at his home in Pangnirtung, surrounded by his family. Few Inuit have lived such a long and abundant life. And in its final chapter, he received thanks and honour from his country and from the community he loved and served.

Etuangat's obituary was printed in the *Nunatsiaq News*, Iqaluit, on January 19, 1996. Otto Schaefer received the news in a phone call from an old Pangnirtung colleague, Vera Roberts. Etuangat and Otto had bidden farewell to each other many times before; this was the time for a final *Tabawutit* (good-bye) to his friend of 41 years.

44
Living Memories

On Saturday, September 21, 1996 Otto Schaefer took me on a tour of his home in Edmonton. Designed by the Schaefers in Bavarian style and built in 1966, it had obviously once rung with the laughter and cheery voices of several children. Now it seemed very quiet and still. But on every shelf and window sill, in every corner, and on every wall were pictures and artifacts that told the story of those halcyon years in the North.

We first visited the upstairs bedrooms, each of which had a door opening onto a "wraparound" type of Swiss balcony. In the room where Didi breathed her last, we saw Otto's much-cherished picture of her, backpack firmly in place, hiking up past Staircase Falls towards Summit Lake in rugged Auyittuq National Park. Looking at this special picture, Otto commented that she was cheerful and thankful right up until the end, "much more philosophical and wiser and with a much more positive attitude than I have ever had."

Down the hall were the rooms of the children, long since grown up. On the walls of the room shared by Lothar and Alfred were pictures of mountain scenes, skiing, and kayaking. One picture showed Alfred astride his heavily laden bike, ready to pedal to the next destination during his five-year tour of Africa. Another showed the Columbia Icefields photographed from his hang glider 300 metres up.

All three of the girls' rooms displayed a large poster of the endangered wolf, bearing the caption "Just let it be!" The walls of Heidi's room were covered with pictures and posters of lions, horses, skiing and whitewater canoeing scenes. The clothes in her closet and the small items on her desk remained as they had been at the time of her death in December 1988.

Walking down the staircase, we suddenly faced a large picture: it depicted the wrinkled but animated face of a venerable Inuit patriarch from the Patliq area northwest of Arviat. Nearby was the no less revealing pencil sketch of a young mother and child. This was a self-portrait by Selena Iruk, who had assisted Hildes and Schaefer during their surveys at Igloolik and Hall Beach.

Except for one wall, almost every available inch of wall space in the bright and spacious living room was filled with books, pictures, and magnificent artifacts and relics from the Arctic. But the piano stood in isolation. In my mind I could picture Otto's friend from Siberia, the ebullient Kaznacheyev, who had once sat at the keyboard and filled the room with his loud, mellifluous baritone voice.

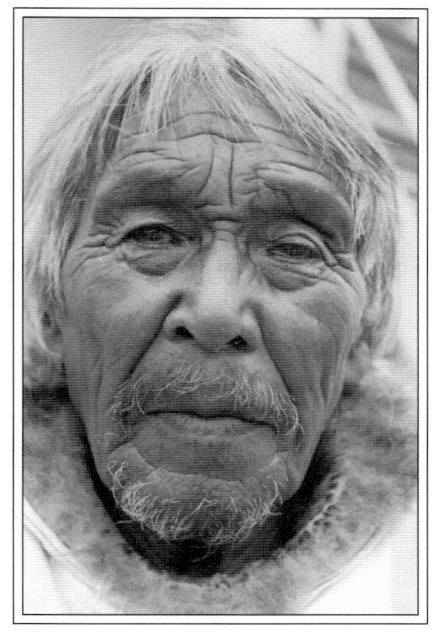

Inuit patriarch on board the C.D. Howe in August 1964.

As if to bring things down to earth, on the floor at one end lay an oblong seal oil lamp, shaped and hollowed from a flat soapstone. I wondered what Inuit wife had slept beside that lamp, waking up every half hour to trim or adjust the line of Arctic cotton wicks or swirl the oil around.

Along the wide windowsills and on shelves by the fireplace I saw several of the celebrated Inuit soapstone carvings, works of art of amazing beauty. One in particular caught my eye: that of a mother bowed down with the weight of two infants in the *amauti* (baby pouch) on her back inside her parka. The reason for her heavy burden was only too clear: one of the infants was sucking on a bottle. The carver from Inukjuak on

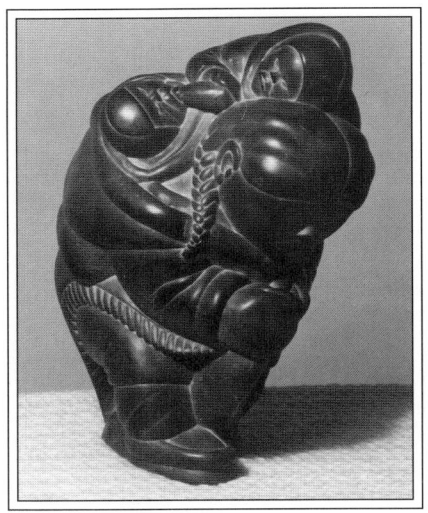

Soapstone carving by Simionie from Inukjuak (Port Harrison), showing a mother burdened by two infants. Purchased by Otto Schaefer in Ottawa in 1967.

the east coast of Hudson Bay obviously understood the problem that Otto had battled for many years.

The large, heavy soapstone carving of a delivery scene showed how family and friends gather around to help the mother-to-be. In fact, the two young unmarried men supporting her arms and shoulders were there to learn about childbirth for the time when they would be needed.

Two whale bone carvings rested on a shelf nearby. In one, a miniature igloo had been made of tiny flake-like squares of bone the thickness of a potato chip. The lead-like weight of another, somewhat larger carving of whale bone surprised me, until Otto explained that whales need heavy bones to counteract the buoyancy of hundreds of pounds of blubber.

One of the most exquisite works of art was a series of fine carvings along the entire length of a caribou antler. On the finely polished antler had been implanted tiny, intricately carved ivory objects from hunting scenes: a caribou swimming, a man in his kayak, a hunter poised by a seal's breathing hole with spear in hand. It was a magnificent creation.

I saw some of the distinctive Inuit prints. The printmaking technique had been perfected and popularized under the guidance of James Houston in Cape Dorset and Salluit. As Otto explained, the design is created by carving the images in stone and then printing on fabric and paper using Chinese ink.

One print showed a hunter, cut adrift on an ice floe, saving his life by making a sail of sealskin and using the wind to take him back to shore. Another showed a circular stone trap used to catch Arctic char in their pre-winter migration upstream to inland lakes. When a number of fish have been caught in the trap, the people go in with their spears.

Occupying most of one wall was a magnificent rug of polar bear fur. This creature had once roamed the southeast part of Cumberland Peninsula, a relatively uninhabited area where "the polar bear reigns supreme."

Over the fireplace I stood for some time admiring the tightly spiralled tusk of a narwhal, two metres long. Otto informed me that the actual function of this massive, unicorn-like structure, said to be an elongated canine tooth, is not really understood. The whale uses it not as an aggressive weapon, but possibly for extracting clams from the sea bed. In another area I saw the cervical vertebra of a beluga whale, a cousin of the narwhal. The projecting bone ends had been carved and polished into walrus heads.

One of the most interesting of the relics was the tip of a harpoon made of ivory from a walrus tusk. Estimated to be over 600 years old, it had been found under the moss at Resolute Bay on Cornwallis Island in the High Arctic.

Down in the recreation room, Otto showed me an arresting painting that depicted an Inuit myth or legend. The central figure, a dog, is "speaking" to a man armed with bow and arrow. To the dog had been transferred the living soul of the hunter's father, killed some time before by the three other figures in the painting. The dog/father orders the young hunter to avenge his death and to shoot arrows at the others. If they fire back at him, the dog will jump up and intercept the arrows. In the scene, one man is running away, another lies with an arrow through his heart, and the third is about ready to pay the price for his villainy.

In another room I saw one of Otto's favourite pictures, one he had taken of the bay at Pangnirtung at mid-afternoon in late November. Over the hills, the whole western sky is aglow with crimson and gold. Like autumn leaves whose beauty reaches a climax just before they fall, the sun too was falling out of sight and would remain so for a month and a half.

In a separate room, we opened the door of a closet full of clothes from the past. We took off the rack one of Didi's Aklavik parkas made of soft reindeer skins with a collar of wolverine fur. I wondered about Otto's parka that he wore so often on dog team trips at Pangnirtung. I learned that it had been left behind: "too stained and worn for civilization," he said. Also in the closet hung a fine sealskin jacket, a gift from the wife of the special constable at Pangnirtung. The ivory buttons, carved in the form of a face, were the work of Etuangat.

In another room I saw the carving of a hunter and a harpooned walrus, a fine piece of handiwork, made for Otto by a friend from Hudson Bay.

We bypassed the study twice until I specifically requested that we go in. The desk scattered with papers and a half-filled page in the typewriter spoke of a man still at work. Memoirs, some in German, others in English, lay in piles.

On the walls of this room, where I suspect visitors were rarely invited, I saw numerous framed honours and awards, some of which I knew little or nothing about. For example, there was his 1976 Alberta Achievement Award "in recognition of excellence in northern medical research, with best wishes and congratulations from the people and government of Alberta," signed by Premier Peter Lougheed.

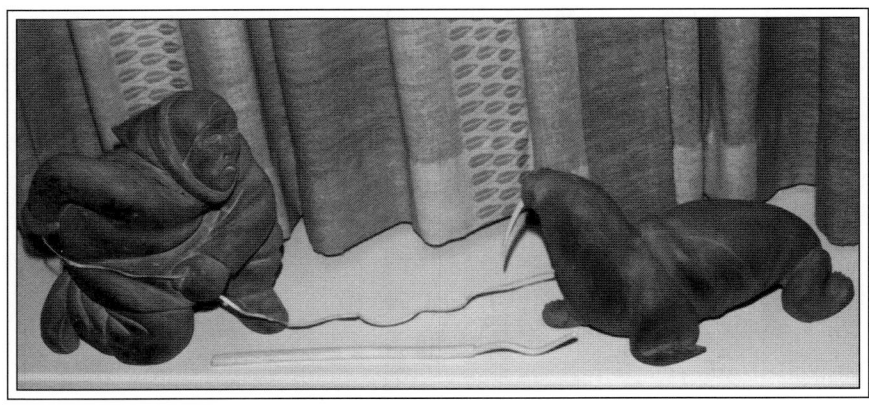

Hunter and harpooned walrus carving made for Otto by Mosesie.

There also hung the framed Doctor of Science Honorary Award "in recognition of distinguished academic achievement" received from the University of Manitoba in 1991.

He showed me a special treasure, the Jack Hildes Medal presented to him by the University of Manitoba in 1987. As the first recipient, he was invited to address the gathering assembled in Winnipeg for the occasion. In his speech, he paid tribute to Hildes, who had launched him on the right path and then became a lifelong friend and collaborator. Along with the medal had come a cheque for $1000, little of which got home because "it was spent on friends in Winnipeg."

I was sorry when our tour had to end—at my request, because time was drawing short. Besides, it was a little hard keeping up with Otto as he scampered up and down stairs and from one room to another. Rarely walking, he still trotted around with the quick, short "ground squirrel" steps that had given him the name *shik-shik* when he and Didi first set foot in the Arctic on that chill January day in 1953.

When I asked what had been the highlight of his life, he replied without hesitation, "Living with Didi in our little white house in Pangnirtung and travelling by dog team around Cumberland Sound and over the mountains to Davis Strait." Life was simple, comforts were few, and hardships many, but somehow "it was idyllic." Nothing could compare with the savage beauty of glacier-lined Pangnirtung Fiord with its lacy network of creeks and waterfalls, soaring rugged cliffs, and mountains. No wonder Didi called it "the embodiment of paradise."

But it was more than the scenery, the spectacular and wild terrain. More than anything else, it was the people, his co-workers in the hospital and the community and his Inuit friends, that endeared Pangnirtung to him. He would always cherish the memory of these friends. Asked for his own personal views of the Cumberland Sound Inuit, he said he simply could not improve on the words used by Franz Boas in 1883:

The kindness and sensitivity of the Inuit, the sympathetic tact that they demonstrated in their personal relationships, gave proof that inner character [herzensbildung was the word he used] was far more

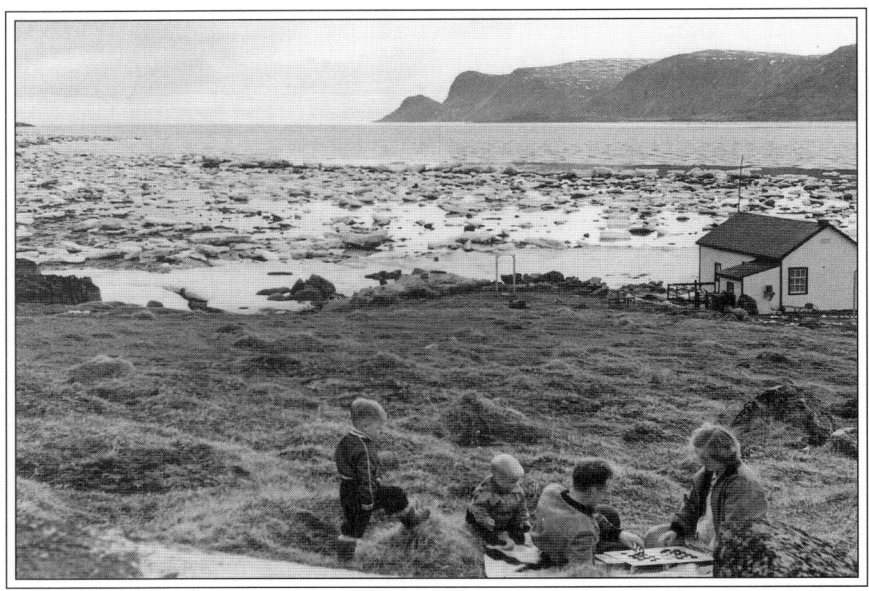

The Schaefers enjoy a warm afternoon on the slopes above their home in Pangnirtung.

significant than the gloss of civilization and learning. (cited in Cole, 1986)

Walking through his home with Otto Schaefer, still slender and trim in his late seventies, I got the feeling that life must be lonely, that all the best days were past. He assured me this was not so, and quoted a verse from a poem by the Chinese poet, Lao Tse, that expressed his true feelings:

> *Bright, glorious days! Don't cry because they're gone,*
> *But smile: rejoice that they have been.*

45
If Otto Schaefer hadn't gone to the Arctic

"CANADA has been lucky to get him," said Dr. Maurice Beare of Otto Schaefer, his colleague for four years at the Charles Camsell Hospital in Edmonton. How does one measure the contribution of a man? And how does one determine the value of that contribution? Did Albert Einstein do more to improve the lot, brighten the life, and widen the horizons of the human race than, say, Elvis Presley? What about Roentgen, who introduced x-rays, or Fleming, who discovered penicillin?

How much were the lives of Native people of the North affected by the work of Otto Schaefer? His sterling record of service to the sick and injured at Aklavik, Pangnirtung, and Whitehorse is undeniable, but service alone has its limitations. Did his work as director of the Northern Medical Research Unit really make any improvement in "their appalling state of health?"

Certainly the breadth and depth of his research—all the way from Old Crow in the Yukon to Cape Dyer on Baffin Island—was astounding. Not only did he study many areas generally ignored by medical authorities of the time, but he often challenged prevailing attitudes and ideas. During his studies of alcohol abuse, for example, he demonstrated that Indians and Inuit metabolize alcohol much more slowly than white people. And Otto Schaefer was one of the first physicians to recognize the foetal alcohol syndrome, in which the newborn suffers brain damage as a consequence of the mother's excessive alcohol intake during pregnancy.

His 110 papers and publications covered an impressive and wide range of subjects. They included the spread of infectious diseases, adaptation to cold, the Inuit "frozen lung," the malnutrition resulting from giving up their traditional diet, the harm of bottle feeding, the changes in the incidence of cancer, the crumbling of the family structure, and the onset of diseases of civilization, to name but a few (Schaefer, 1993).

His writings and addresses extracted from him the utmost in thought and careful preparation. "He was a stickler for accuracy," said one of his associates. Otto once commented that his work on a project that consumed months of his time usually ended up as a few lines in a medical journal that few would read.

Not for a moment did he overlook the need for the practical application of his research studies. He did his best to disseminate his own findings, along with research results from various Canadian and international sources on similar subjects, to all health care workers in the Medical Services Branch. They all got used to getting his "little memos." And he did his best to give radio talks and public addresses and newspaper reports. All this medical and health information he tried to express in simple, nontechnical language.

Whitehorse was not the only place where he ran headlong into opposition, in that case from white pub-keepers who were taking advantage of their Indian patrons. He would not hesitate to condemn a practice that was harmful to Native people, regardless of what the authorities said. He recognized the value of health education, community health, and Native health workers at a time when these were neither medically nor politically fashionable.

Asked for his own assessment of his 32 years working for the people of the North, he had little to say. But he did admit that "some of my observations caused much discussion in scientific as well as public media." He denied having any major role in one of the greatest medical triumphs—the control of tuberculosis—and gave the credit to early identification of open cases, evacuation of the more serious ones, and the use of more effective drugs. He failed to mention that right from the early Aklavik days, he was involved in caring for patients with TB and did some original studies on INH (Isonicotinic Acid Hydrazide), one of the more effective drugs.

Often he had felt encouraged. After he gave a talk on nutrition and good health practices, audience members would come up to express appreciation and their hope that young people were getting his message. When asked if the many gifts that had come to him were an expression of this gratitude, he answered, "Maybe, but it's more likely they were gestures of friendship."

A reporter with the *London Free Press* (July 26, 1976) interviewing Otto in 1976 asked: "Is it not true that you are credited with helping bring the epidemic rate of tuberculosis in Indians and Inuit under control?" Otto's reply was that his efforts were not very special.

Does the work of "an internationally known and respected expert in circumpolar health" necessarily benefit the health and life of the people of the North? Gerald Amerongen, former Speaker of the Alberta Legislature and a long-time Schaefer friend, answered without hesitation: "Yes, because his academic research and studies were done specifically to benefit them (the Inuit)."

In support of the practical value of Otto's work, the Canadian Public Health Association in 1982 presented him with the "Ortho Award." The citation included the following:

The quality of his work has won the admiration of researchers both in Canada and abroad.... His studies have invariably had a practical application and his findings have had a significant impact on northern health care delivery. (Ortho Award, 1982:152)

Whatever else might be said, little systematic research had been done on the health of the scattered people of the Canadian North until Otto Schaefer came on the scene. As nurse Kay Dier said of his early days, "Right from the beginning, he had the vision of what could and should be done and tried to gather data in a little book, while doing his regular clinical work."

Years after their association at the Charles Camsell Hospital, Dr. A.M. "Buzz" Edwards, his senior in internal medicine at the time, made these comments:

His immense contribution to Inuit health has been widely recognized. I can't overemphasize his selfless, intense devotion to duty and care of the health problems in the North. He is unique, certainly in North America, as the man with the most experience and personal knowledge of the Inuit. His contribution to their health needs can't be overestimated.

The work of the *Luttakulu* (dear little doctor) had not been in vain.

Appendix
Selected Papers of Otto Schaefer

SCHAEFER, O. 1944. Zur Klinik und Pathogenese Symptomatischer Psychosen bei Nierenkrankheiten. (Clinical manifestation and pathogenesis of symptomatic psychoses in the course of renal disease.) Dissertation for qualification of Doctorate in Medicine at the University of Heidelberg, Germany. 81 p.

DELIUS, L., and SCHAEFER, O. 1950. Zur Erorterung der Begriffsbestimmung und der Therapie des "Myocard-schadens." (To the definition and therapy of "Myocardio-damage.") Der Landzart 26(11): 2–5.

SCHAEFER, O. 1957. Erlebnisse und Erfahrungen eines deutschen Arztes im hohen Norden Kanadas. (Experiences and observations of a German physician in the far north of Canada.) Münchener Medizinische Wochenschrift 99(34):1208–1213.

SCHAEFER, O. 1957. Eingeborenen-Medizin bei Indianern und Eskimos im ussersten Norden Kanadas. (Aboriginal medicine practised by Indians and Eskimos in the far north of Canada.) Münchener Medizinische Wochenschrift 99(48):1833–1835.

SCHAEFER, O. 1958. Arteriosklerose-Frage in Eskimos. (Concerning arteriosclerotic manifestations in Eskimos.) Münchener Medizinische Wochenschrift 100(32):1202.

SCHAEFER, O. 1959. Zur Arteriosklerose-Frage in Eskimos (Concerning arteriosclerosis in Eskimos – Dietary factors, the protective role of arctic sea-mammal fats.) Münchener Medizinische Wochenschrift 101:250.

SCHAEFER, O. 1959. Neoplasmen bei kanadischen Eskimos. (Neoplastic diseases in Canadian Eskimos.) Münchener Medizinische Wochenschrift 191:984.

SCHAEFER, O. 1959. Medical observations and problems in the Canadian Arctic. Parts I and II. Canadian Medical Association Journal 81:248–253 and 386–393.

SCHAEFER, O. 1960. Letter to the Editor: Incidence of neoplastic diseases in Canadian Eskimos. Canadian Medical Association Journal 82:280–281.

SCHAEFER, O. 1960. Familial occurrence of abnormal placentation and fetal malformations observed in Baffin Island Eskimos. Canadian Medical Association Journal 83:437–438.

SCHAEFER, O. 1962. Alcohol withdrawal syndrome in a newborn infant of a Yukon Indian mother. Canadian Medical Association Journal 87:1333–1334.

SCHAEFER, O. 1964. Nutritional problems in the Eskimos. Canadian Nutritional Notes 20(8):85–90.

SCHAEFER, O. 1966. Letter to the Editor: Accidental deaths among British Columbia Indians. Canadian Medical Association Journal 94:684–685.

SCHAEFER, O. 1966. Pulmonary miliary calcifications and histoplasmin sensitivity in Canadian Eskimos. Canadian Journal of Public Health 57:410–412.

SCHAEFER, O. 1968. Glycosuria and diabetes mellitus in Canadian Eskimos. Canadian Medical Association Journal 99:201–206.

SCHAEFER, O. 1968. Glucose tolerance testing in Canadian Eskimos: A preliminary report and a hypothesis. Canadian Medical Association Journal 99:252–262.

SCHAEFER, O. 1969. Carbohydrate metabolism in Eskimos. Archives of Environmental Health 18:144–147.

SCHAEFER, O. 1969. Letter to the Editor: Cancer of the breast and lactation. Canadian Medical Association Journal 100:625–626.

SCHAEFER, O. 1969. Diet, physical activity, blood lipids and incidence of cardiovascular abnormalities in elderly male Eskimos of the Canadian Eastern Arctic. Paper presented at the 8th International Congress of Nutrition in Prague, Czechoslovakia, 28 August – 5 September, 1969.

CONWAY, D.J., and SCHAEFER, O. 1969. Nutritional anemia in the Eastern Arctic. Scientific exhibit at the annual meeting of the Canadian

Pediatric Society, Ottawa, Ontario. Also presented as a paper at the 8th International Congress of Nutrition in Prague, Czechoslovakia, 28 August – 5 September, 1969.

SCHAEFER, O. 1970. Pre-and post-natal growth acceleration and increased sugar consumption in Canadian Eskimos. Canadian Medical Association Journal 103:1059–1068.

RONALD, A.R., ALTOSE, M.D., HILDES, J.A., and SCHAEFER, O. 1970. Meningococcal carrier surveys at Baker Lake, NWT. Canadian Journal of Public Health 61:80.

SCHAEFER, O. 1971. Otitis media and bottle-feeding: An epidemiological study of infant feeding habits and incidence of recurrent and chronic middle ear disease in Canadian Eskimos. Canadian Journal of Public Health 62(6):478–489.

SCHAEFER, O. 1971. Physiological and pathological effects of nutritional changes in the Canadian Arctic. Paper presented at the 2nd International Symposium on Circumpolar Health in Oulu, Finland.

SCHAEFER, O. 1971. When the Eskimo comes to town. Nutrition Today 6(6):8–16.

FENNA, D., MIX, L., SCHAEFER, O., and GILBERT, J.A.L. 1971. Ethanol metabolism in various racial groups. Canadian Medical Association Journal 105:472–475.

JEANES, C.W.L., SCHAEFER, O., and EIDUS, L. 1972. Inactivation of isoniazid by Canadian Eskimos and Indians. Canadian Medical Association Journal 106:331–335.

SCHAEFER, O., CROCKFORD, P.M., and ROMANOWSKI, B. 1972. Normalization effect of preceding protein meals on "diabetic" oral glucose tolerance in Eskimos. Canadian Medical Association Journal 107:733–738.

SCHAEFER, O. 1973. The changing health picture in the Canadian North. Canadian Journal of Ophthalmology 8:196–204.

SCHAEFER, O. 1973. Vigorous exercise and coronary heart disease. The Lancet, April 14:840.

SCHAEFER, O. 1973. Discussion of the alcohol problem in the Native population of the Canadian North and proposed steps to deal with the problem. In: Science and the North: A seminar on guidelines for scientific activities in northern Canada. Ottawa: Information Canada. 52–55.

HILDES, J.A., and SCHAEFER, O. 1973. Health of Igloolik Eskimos and changes with urbanization. Journal of Human Evolution 2:241–246.

JEANES, C.W.L., SCHAEFER, O., and EIDUS, L. 1973. Comparative blood levels and metabolism of INH and an INH-matrix preparation in fast and slow inactivators. Canadian Medical Association Journal 109:483–487.

SCHAEFER, O. 1974. Otitis media in Eskimos. Pediatrics 54:52.

SCHAEFER, O. 1974. Unmet needs of Canadian Indian and Eskimo children. In: Dunn, R.G., ed. First Canadian Ross Conference on Pediatric Research. Montreal: Ross Lab. 382–388.

SCHAEFER, O. 1974. The relative roles of diet and physical activity on blood lipids and obesity. American Heart Journal 88:673–674.

EIDUS, L., HODGKIN, M.M., SCHAEFER, O., and JESSAMINE, A.G. 1974. Distribution of isoniazid inactivators determined in Eskimos and Canadian college students by urine test. Revue Canadienne de Biologie 33:117–123.

EIDUS, L., and SCHAEFER, O. 1974. Tuberculosis treatment for "rapid" metabolizers of isoniazid: A problem particular in Canadian Indians and Eskimos. Modern Medicine of Canada 29(1):18–20.

HERXHEIMER, H., and SCHAEFER, O. 1974. Asthma in Canadian Eskimos. New England Medical Journal 291:1419.

SCHAEFER, O., HILDES, J.A., GREIDANUS, P., and LEUNG, D. 1974. Regional sweating in Eskimos compared to Caucasians. Canadian Journal of Physiology and Pharmacology 52:960–965.

SCHAEFER, O. 1975. Food resources and changing dietary patterns of the Eskimo child. In: Haworth, J.C., ed. Second Ross Conference on Pediatric Research: Nutrition of Indian and Eskimo children. Toronto, Ontario, November 1974. Montreal: Ross Laboratories. 19–22.

SCHAEFER, O. 1975. Health-related aspects of transitional Inuit society. University of Manitoba Medical Journal 45(3):98–103.

SCHAEFER, O. 1975. Eskimo personality and society—Yesterday and today. Arctic 28(2):87–91.

ELLESTAD-SAYED, J., HILDES, J.A., SCHAEFER, O., and LOBBAN, M.D. 1975. Twenty-four hour urinary excretion of vitamins, minerals and nitrogen by Eskimos. American Journal of Clinical Nutrition 28:1402–1407.

HARLEY, C.H., SCOTT, G.W., and SCHAEFER, O. 1975. Pulmonary echinococcosis in northwestern Canada. Paper presented at the annual meeting of the Royal College of Physicians and Surgeons, Winnipeg, Manitoba, January 1975.

HILDES, J.A., ELLESTAD-SAYED, J., and SCHAEFER, O. 1975. A health profile of the Iglooligmiut. Paper presented at the annual meeting of the Canadian Association of Physical Anthropologists, Winnipeg, Manitoba, October 1975.

SAYED, J.E., HILDES, J.A., and SCHAEFER, O. 1975. Nutrition of the Canadian Eskimo child. In: Haworth, J.C., ed. Second Ross Conference on Pediatric Research: Nutrition of Indian and Eskimo children. Toronto, Ontario, November 1974. Montreal: Ross Laboratories. 35–38.

SCHAEFER, O. 1976. Socio-cultural change and health in Canadian Inuit. In: Tremblay, M.A., ed. Les Facettes de l'Identité Amerindienne—The patterns of Amerindian identity. Laval, Quebec: Les Presses de l'Université. 279–300.

EIDUS, L., SCHAEFER, O., and HODGKIN, M.M. 1976. Methodology and results of phenotyping isoniazid inactivators In: Shephard, R.J., and Itoh, S., eds. Circumpolar Health. Proceedings of the 3rd International Symposium of Circumpolar Health, Yellowknife, NWT, 8–11 July 1974. Toronto: University of Toronto Press. 342–348.

HENDZEL, M., SAYED, J.E., SCHAEFER, O., and HILDES, J.A. 1976. Mercury content of Iglooligmiut hair. In: Shephard, R.J., and Itoh, S., eds. Circumpolar Health. Proceedings of the 3rd International Symposium of Circumpolar Health, Yellowknife, NWT, 8–11 July 1974. Toronto: University of Toronto Press. 658–663.

HILDES, J.A., SCHAEFER, O., SAYED, J.E., FITZGERALD, E.J., and KOCH, E.A. 1976. Chronic lung disease and cardiovascular consequences in Iglooligmiut. In: Shephard, R.J., and Itoh, S., eds. Circumpolar Health. Proceedings of the 3rd International Symposium of Circumpolar Health,

Yellowknife, NWT, 8–11 July 1974. Toronto: University of Toronto Press. 327–331.

HODGKIN, M.M., EIDUS, L., SCHAEFER, O., POLLAK, B., and LEUNG, D. 1976. Intermittent chemotherapy of tuberculosis patients rapidly inactivating isoniazid. In: Shephard, R.J., and Itoh, S., eds. Circumpolar Health. Proceedings of the 3rd International Symposium of Circumpolar Health, Yellowknife, NWT, 8–11 July 1974. Toronto: University of Toronto Press. 348–353.

SAYED, J.E., HILDES, J.A., and SCHAEFER, O. 1976. Biochemical indices of nutrition of the Iglooligmiut. In: Shephard, R.J., and Itoh, S., eds. Circumpolar Health. Proceedings of the 3rd International Symposium of Circumpolar Health, Yellowknife, NWT, 8–11 July 1974. Toronto: University of Toronto Press. 130–134.

SAYED, J.E., HILDES, J.A., and SCHAEFER, O. 1976. Feeding practices and growth of Igloolik infants In: Shephard, R.J., and Itoh, S., eds. Circumpolar Health. Proceedings of the 3rd International Symposium of Circumpolar Health, Yellowknife, NWT, 8–11 July 1974. Toronto: University of Toronto Press. 254–259.

SAYED, H., SAYED, J., HILDES, J.A., and SCHAEFER, O. 1976. Commentary: Deficiency of secretory IgA in Eskimo saliva. In: Shephard, R.J., and Itoh, S., eds. Circumpolar Health. Proceedings of the 3rd International Symposium of Circumpolar Health, Yellowknife, NWT, 8–11 July 1974. Toronto: University of Toronto Press. 221.

SCHAEFER, O., HILDES, J.A., GREIDANUS, P., and LEUNG, D. 1976. Regional sweating in Eskimos and Caucasians. In: Shephard, R.J., and Itoh, S., eds. Circumpolar Health. Proceedings of the 3rd International Symposium of Circumpolar Health, Yellowknife, NWT, 8–11 July 1974. Toronto: University of Toronto Press. 46–49.

SCHAEFER, O., HILDES, J.A., MEDD, L.M., and CAMERON, D.G. 1976. The changing pattern of neoplastic disease in Canadian Eskimos. In: Shephard, R.J., and Itoh, S., eds. Circumpolar Health. Proceedings of the 3rd International Symposium of Circumpolar Health, Yellowknife, NWT, 8–11 July 1974. Toronto: University of Toronto Press. 277–283.

SCHAEFER, O., and METAYER, M. 1976. Eskimo personality and society – yesterday and today. In: Shephard, R.J., and Itoh, S., eds. Circumpolar Health. Proceedings of the 3rd International Symposium of Circumpolar Health, Yellowknife, NWT, 8–11 July 1974. Toronto: University of Toronto Press. 469–479.

SCHAEFER, O. 1977. Changing dietary patterns in the Canadian North: Health, social and economic consequences. Journal of the Canadian Dietetic Association 38:17–25.

SCHAEFER, O. 1977. When the Eskimo comes to town. A follow-up. Nutrition Today May/June:21–23.

SCHAEFER, O. 1977. Are Eskimos more or less obese than other Canadians? A comparison of skinfold thickness and ponderal index in Canadian Eskimos. American Journal of Clinical Nutrition 30:1623–1628.

SCHAEFER, O. 1978. Health in our time? The Canadian Nurse 74:32–36.

HOPPNER, K., McLAUGHLIN, J.M., SHAH, B.G., THOMPSON, J.N., BEARE-ROGERS, J., ELLESTAD-SAYED, J., and SCHAEFER, O. 1978. Nutrient levels of some foods of Eskimos from Arctic Bay, N.W.T., Canada. Journal of the American Dietetic Association 73(3):257–260.

SCHAEFER, O. 1979. Aetiology of appendicitis: Sharp increases in incidennce when Eskimos switch from traditional carnivore to imported carbohydrate diet. British Medical Journal (May):1215.

SCHAEFER, O. 1979. When breastfeeding declines. Changes in infant feeding practices in the Canadian Eskimos, social and health consequences. Presented at La Leche League International, Atlanta, Georgia. Summarized in La Leche League News 21:88–89.

SCHAEFER, O. 1980. Interaction of diseases, nutrition and demography in Canadian Inuit during the last generation. Paper presented at the 2nd Inuit Studies Conference, 15–18 September, Quebec City, Quebec.

SCHAEFER, O. 1980. Diet, blood lipids and coronary disease. "Lo-the poor Eskimo!" American Heart Journal 100:944–945.

SCHAEFER, O., EATON, R.D.P., TIMMERMANS, F.J.W., and HILDES, J.A. 1980. Respiratory function impairment and cardiopulmonary consequences in long-time residents of the Canadian Arctic. Canadian Medical Association Journal 123:997–1004.

SCHAEFER, O., and STECKLE, J. 1980. Dietary habits and nutritional base of Native populations of the Northwest Territories. Yellowknife, N.W.T.: Science Advisory Board of the Northwest Territories, Canada.

SCHAEFER, O., TIMMERMANS, F.J.W., EATON, R.D.P., and MATTHEWS, A.R. 1980. General and nutritional health in two Eskimo populations at different stages of acculturation. Canadian Journal of Public Health 71:397–405.

SCHAEFER, O. 1981. Growth standards in different ethnic groups. The Lancet, January 10:101.

SCHAEFER, O. 1981. Eskimos (Inuit). In: Trowell, H.C., Burkitt, D.P., and Arnold, E., eds. Western diseases: Their emergence and prevention. 113–128.

SCHAEFER, O. 1981. Changing morbidity and mortality patterns in Canadian Inuit. Chronic Diseases in Canada 2(2):12–18.

SCHAEFER, O. 1981. Observations on the mortality of Alberta Indians. Chronic Diseases in Canada 2(3):37.

SCHAEFER, O. 1981. Cancer mortality by ethnic group in B.C. Chronic Diseases in Canada 2(3):12.

ROMANOWSKI, E., and SCHAEFER, O. 1981. Alcoholic liver cirrhosis in Indian and non-Indian patients in Charles Camsell Hospital, 1950–1980. Chronic Diseases in Canada 2(2):19–20.

SCHAEFER, O. 1982. Knud Rasmussen Memorial Lecture. Ethnology, demography and medicine in the Arctic. In: Harvald, B., and Hart Hansen, J.P., eds. Circumpolar Health 81. Proceedings of the 5th International Symposium on Circumpolar Health, Copenhagen, 9–13 August 1981. Copenhagen: Nordic Council for Arctic Medical Research. 187–193.

SCHAEFER, O. 1982. Human adaptation: Health and disease. Transactions of the Royal Society of Canada, Series 4, Vol. 20:418–427.

SCHAEFER, O. 1982. Review of changes in nutritional habits and nutritional resources in northern Canadian Natives and related health consequences. In: Praamsma, K., and Komerchuk, K., eds. Scientific Papers of the 73rd Canadian Public Health Association Conference: Environment, Lifestyles, Heredity, June 1982, Yellowknife, N.W.T. 222–228.

SCHAEFER, O. 1982. The changing epidemiological picture in the Canadian North: A reflection of the interplay of environment, lifestyle and heredity. In: Praamsma, K., and Komerchuk, K., eds. Scientific Papers of the 73rd Canadian Public Health Association Conference: Environment, Lifestyles, Heredity, June 1982, Yellowknife, N.W.T. 633–647.

BENDER, T.R., LANIER, A.P., HALL, D.B., NIELSEN, N.H., HART-HANSEN, J.P., and SCHAEFER, O. 1982. The evolution of cancer as an important health problem for Eskimos. In: Harvald, B., and Hart Hansen, J.P., eds. Circumpolar Health 81. Proceedings of the 5th International Symposium on Circumpolar Health, Copenhagen, 9–13 August 1981. Copenhagen: Nordic Council for Arctic Medical Research. 258–264.

HILDES, J.A., and SCHAEFER, O. 1982. Inuit malignancy update: The changing picture of neoplastic disease in the Canadian Western and Central Arctic, 1950–80. In: Praamsma, K., and Komerchuk, K., eds. Scientific Papers of the 73rd Canadian Public Health Association Conference: Environment, Lifestyles, Heredity, June 1982, Yellowknife, N.W.T. 206–210.

LARKE, R.P.B., EATON, R.D.P., and SCHAEFER, O. 1982. Epidemiology of hepatitis B in the Canadian Arctic. In: Harvald, B., and Hart-Hansen, J.P., eds. Circumpolar Health 81. Proceedings of the 5th International Symposium on Circumpolar Health, Copenhagen, 9–13 August 1981. Copenhagen: Nordic Council for Arctic Medical Research. 401–406.

SCHAEFER, O., and SPADY, D.W. 1982. Changing trends in infant feeding patterns in the Northwest Territories 1973–1979. Canadian Journal of Public Health 73:304–309.

SPADY, D.W., COVILL, F.J., HOBART, C.W., SCHAEFER, O., and TASKER, R.S. 1982. Between two worlds: Report of the Infant Mortality and Morbidity Study (PIMMS) 1973/74. Occasional Publication No. 16. Edmonton: Boreal Institute, University of Alberta.

SCHAEFER, O. 1983. Psycho-social problems experienced by Native population groups in the Canadian Arctic involved in resource development. Canadian Journal of Community Mental Health, Special Suppl. 1:53–55.

SCHAEFER, O. 1984. Adoption and lactation practices of Canadian Inuit. Canadian Journal of Public Health 75:324.

SCHAEFER, O. 1984. Nutrition and health: Impact of changing dietary habits. In: Steckle, J. Northern foodcosts. Ottawa: Health and Welfare Canada.

SCHAEFER, O. 1984. Medical research in remote areas with isolated populations—Needs, benefits and limitations. In: Sarsfield, P., ed. Lectures in community medicine. St. John's, Newfoundland: Memorial University. 12–23.

HILDES, J.A., and SCHAEFER, O. 1984. The changing picture of neoplastic disease in the western and central Canadian Arctic (1950–1980). Canadian Medical Association Journal 130:25–32.

SCHAEFER, O. 1985. Medical research in remote northern areas and isolated populations: Needs, benefits and limitations. In: Fortuine, R., ed. Circumpolar Health 84. Proceedings of the Sixth International Symposium on Circumpolar Health, Anchorage, Alaska, 13–18 May 1984. Seattle: University of Washington Press. 11–16.

CARSON, J.B., POSTL, B.D., SPADY, D., and SCHAEFER, O. 1985. Lower respiratory tract infections among Canadian Inuit children. In: Fortuine, R., ed. Circumpolar Health 84. Proceedings of the Sixth International Symposium on Circumpolar Health, Anchorage, Alaska, 13–18 May 1984. Seattle: University of Washington Press. 226–228.

POSTL, B.D., CARSON, J.B., SPADY, D., and SCHAEFER, O. 1985. Northwest Territories Perinatal and Infant Morbidity and Mortality Study: Follow-up 1982 I. Utilization, morbidity and mortality. In: Fortuine, R., ed. Circumpolar Health 84. Proceedings of the Sixth International Symposium on Circumpolar Health. Anchorage, Alaska, 13–18 May 1984. Seattle: University of Washington Press. 125–128.

POSTL, B., CARSON, J., SPADY, D. and SCHAEFER, O. 1985. Northwest Territories Perinatal and Infant Morbidity and Mortality Study: Follow-up 1982 II. Physical examination. In: Fortuine, R., ed. Circumpolar Health 84. Proceedings of the Sixth International Symposium on Circumpolar Health. Anchorage, Alaska, 13–18 May 1984. Seattle: University of Washington Press. 129–133.

SCHAEFER, O. 1986. The impact of culture on breastfeeding patterns. Journal of Perinatology 6(1):62–65.

SCHAEFER, O. 1986. Adverse reactions to drugs and metabolic problems perceived in northern Indians and Eskimos. In: Kalow, W., Goedde, H.W., and Agarwal, D.P., eds. Ethnic differences in reactions to drugs and xenobiotics. New York: Alan R. Liss. 77–83.

SCHAEFER, O. 1986. Cancer of the cervix in Canadian Indians and Inuit— A preventable epidemic. Chronic Diseases in Canada 7(1):2–3.

SCHAEFER, O. 1987. Carbohydrate metabolism in Indians and Inuit. In: Young, T.K., ed. Diabetes in the Canadian Native population. Toronto: Canadian Diabetes Association. 77–84.

SCHAEFER, O. 1988. Comment on "Acculturation and health in the highlands of Papua, New Guinea: Dissent on diversity, diets and development," by G. Dennett and J. Connell. Current Anthropology 29(2):286–287.

SCHAEFER, O. 1988. Native people, health. In: Marsh, J.H., ed. Canadian Encyclopedia, Vol. 3. 2nd ed. Edmonton: Hurtig Publishers. 1452–1453.

SCHAEFER, O. 1988. Contribution to the Panel on Arctic Health. In: Linderholm, H., Backman, C., Broadbent, N., and Joelsson, I., eds. Circumpolar Health 87. Proceedings of the 7th International Congress on Circumpolar Health, Umeå, Sweden, 8–12 June 1987. Oulu: Nordic Council for Arctic Medical Research. 31–33.

SCHAEFER, O., and HILDES, J.A. 1989. Inuit cancer register 1950–1980. In: Parkin, D.M., ed. World Health Organization. Lyon, France. 159–163.

SCHAEFER, O. 1991. *Luttamuit* (Doctor's people) and "old wives' tales"— Their unrecognized value in medicine. In: Postl, B.D., Gilbert, P., Goodwill, J., Moffatt, M.E.K., O'Neil, J.D., Sarsfield, P.A., and Young, T.K., eds. Circumpolar Health 90. Proceedings of the 8th International Congress on Circumpolar Health, Whitehorse, Yukon, 20–25 May 1990. Winnipeg: University of Manitoba Press. 8–11.

SCHAEFER, O. 1994. Changing health picture of Inuit and Indians in the Northwest Territories from the 1950s to the 1980s. Annals of the College of Physicians and Surgeons of Canada 27(2):109–113.

References

ALIKUT, G. 1986. Fall of the wild. Chicago Tribune Magazine (November 2):16.

BOAS, F. 1885. Baffin-Land: Geographische Ergebnisse einer in den Jahren 1883 und 1884 ausgeführten Forschungsreise. Petermanns Mitteilungen, Suppl. 80. 100 p.

———. 1888. The Central Eskimo. Washington, D.C.: Bureau of Ethnology, Smithsonian Institution.

BRETT, H.B. 1969. A synopsis of northern medical history. Canadian Medical Association Journal 100:521–525.

COLE, D. 1986. Franz Boas in Baffin Land. The Beaver 66(4) (August/September):6.

CONWAY, F.J., and SCHAEFER, O. 1969. Nutritional anemia in the Eastern Arctic. Paper presented at the Eighth International Congress of Nutrition, 28 August – 5 September 1969, Prague, Czechoslovakia.

DODGE, D.G. 1989. Heidi Schaefer: She died in the mountains where she loved to be. Parks and Wilderness (Spring 1989):6.

FARB, P. 1968. Man's rise to civilization as shown by the Indians of North America from primeval times to the coming of the industrial state. New York: E.P. Dutton and Co.

FENNA, D., MIX, L., SCHAEFER, O., and GILBERT, J.A.L. 1971. Ethanol metabolism in various racial groups. Canadian Medical Association Journal 105:472–475.

HALLIDAY, H.A. 1995. Rescue mission. The Beaver 75:2 (April/May):14–25.

HARPER, K. 1997. Pangnirtung. In: The 1998 Nunavut Handbook: Travelling in Canada's Arctic. Iqaluit: Nortext Multimedia Inc. 303–310.

HICKS, W. 1972. The good life is hard on the Eskimos. The Canadian Magazine (October 28):22–24.

INDIAN AND NORTHERN AFFAIRS CANADA. 1985. Communiqué: Northern Science Award Presented in Ottawa, December 10, 1985.

KENYON, W.A. 1975. Tokens of possession: The northern voyages of Martin Frobisher. Toronto: Royal Ontario Museum. 164 p.

LEARMONTH, L.A. 1966. Postscript to death in the Arctic. Maclean's Magazine (September 3):31.

MARSH, J.H. 1988. Mackenzie River. In: Marsh, J.H., ed. The Canadian Encyclopedia, Vol. 2. 2nd ed. Edmonton: Hurtig Publishers. 1272–1273.

MOUNTFIELD, D. 1974. A history of polar exploration. London and Toronto: Hamlyn.

MOWAT, F. 1966. The Executioners. Maclean's Magazine (July 2):7–26.

MÜLLER-WILLE, L., ed. 1998. Franz Boas among the Inuit of Baffin Island 1883–1884: Journals and Letters. Translated by William Barr. Toronto: University of Toronto Press. 298 p.

MUSSELL, B. 1976. Circumpolar Health: Keynote address. In: Shephard, R.J., and Itoh, S., eds. Circumpolar Health. Proceedings of the 3rd International Symposium of Circumpolar Health, Yellowknife, NWT, 8–11 July 1974. Toronto: University of Toronto Press. 3–7.

NEATBY, L.H. 1958. In quest of the North West Passage. Toronto: Longman, Green and Co.

ORTHO AWARD. 1982. Ortho Award/Prix Ortho. Canadian Journal of Public Health 73:152.

POOL, A. 1988. Gjoa Haven. In: Marsh, J.H., ed. The Canadian Encyclopedia, Vol. 2. 2nd ed. Edmonton: Hurtig Publishers. 901.

RASMUSSEN, K. 1930. Observations on the intellectual culture of the Caribou Eskimos. Translated by W. Worster and W.E. Calvart. Report of the Fifth Thule Expedition 1921–24, Vol. 7, No. 2. Copenhagen: Gyldendalske Boghandel.

RCMP (ROYAL CANADIAN MOUNTED POLICE). 1933. The case of "Albert Johnson." Annual Report of the Royal Canadian Mounted Police for the Year ended September 30, 1932. Ottawa: F.A. Acland. 106–110.

RIGBY, B. 1997. Auyuittuq National Park Reserve. In: The 1998 Nunavut Handbook: Travelling in Canada's Arctic. Iqaluit: Nortext Multimedia Inc. 296–299.

SCHAEFER, O. 1953–57. Personal diary. In possession of Otto Schaefer, Edmonton, Alberta.

———. 1959. Medical observations and problems in the Canadian Arctic. Parts I and II. Canadian Medical Association Journal 81:248–253 and 386–393.

———. 1964. Preliminary evaluation of the Eastern Arctic Survey, 1964. Unpublished report to the Director of Medical Services, Department of Health and Welfare, Ottawa, Ontario.

———. 1965. Nutrition and health surveys of Holman Island, Coppermine, Frobisher Bay and Pangnirtung. Unpublished report to the Director of Medical Services, Department of Health and Welfare, Ottawa, Ontario.

———. 1968. Glycosuria and diabetes mellitus in Canadian Eskimos. Canadian Medical Association Journal 99:201–206.

SCHAEFER, O. 1969. Letter to the Editor: Cancer of the breast and lactation. Canadian Medical Association Journal 100:625–626.

———. 1971. When the Eskimo comes to town. Nutrition Today 6(6): 8–16.

———. 1973. The changing health picture in the Canadian North. Canadian Journal of Ophthalmology 8:196–204.

———. 1974. Unmet needs of Canadian Indian and Eskimo children. In: Dunn, R.G., ed. First Canadian Ross Conference on Paediatric Research. Montreal: Ross Lab. 382–388.

———. 1975a. Health-related aspects of transitional Inuit society. Paper presented at the First Churchill Health Conference in March 1975. University of Manitoba Medical Journal 45(3):98–103.

———. 1975b. Intractable diarrhea in Baffin Zone Eskimo infants. Memorandum to Zone Director, Baffin Zone, with distribution of multiple copies.

———. 1982. Knud Rasmussen Memorial Lecture. Ethnology, demography and medicine in the Arctic. In: Harvald, B., and Hart Hansen, J.P., eds. Circumpolar Health 81. Proceedings of the 5th International Symposium on Circumpolar Health, Copenhagen, 9–13 August 1981. Copenhagen: Nordic Council for Arctic Medical Research. 187–193.

———. 1991. *Luttamiut* (Doctor's people) and "old wives' tales": Their unrecognized value in medicine. In: Postl, B.D., Gilbert, P., Goodwill, J., Moffat, M.E.K., O'Neil, J.D., Sarsfield, P.A., and Young, T.K., eds.Circumpolar Health 90. Proceedings of the 8th International Congress on Circumpolar Health, 20–25 May 1990, Whitehorse, Yukon. Winnipeg: University of Manitoba Press. 8–11.

———, ed. 1993. Health problems and health care delivery in the Canadian North: Selected papers of J.A. Hildes and O. Schaefer. Winnipeg: Northern Health Research Unit, Department of Community Health Sciences, The University of Manitoba. 96 p.

———. 1994. Changing health picture of Inuit and Indians in the Northwest Territories from the 1950s to the 1980s. Annals of the College of Physicians and Surgeons of Canada 27(2):109–113.

SCHAEFER, O., and METAYER, M. 1976. Eskimo personality and society – yesterday and today. In: Shephard, R.J., and Itoh, S., eds. Circumpolar Health. Proceedings of the 3rd International Symposium of Circumpolar Health, Yellowknife, NWT, 8–11 July 1974. Toronto: University of Toronto Press. 469–479.

SCHAEFER, O., HILDES, J.A., GREIDANUS, P., and LEUNG, D. 1974. Regional sweating in Eskimos compared to Caucasians. Canadian Journal of Physiology and Pharmacology 52:960–965.

SCHAEFER, O., EATON, R.D.P., TIMMERMANS, F.J.W., and HILDES, J.A. 1980a. Respiratory function impairment and cardiopulmonary consequences in long-time residents of the Canadian Arctic. Canadian Medical Association Journal 123:997–1004.

SCHAEFER, O., TIMMERMANS, F.J.W., EATON, R.D.P., and MATTHEWS, A.R. 1980b. General and nutritional health in two Eskimo populations at different stages of acculturation. Canadian Journal of Public Health 71:397–405.

SERVICE, R.W. 1909. Ballad of the Northern Lights. In: Ballads of a Cheechako. Toronto: William Briggs.

———. 1944. The Law of the Yukon. In: Songs of a Sourdough. Toronto: Ryerson Press.

SHEPHARD, R.J., and ITOH, S. Preface. In: Shephard, R.J., and Itoh, S., eds. Circumpolar Health. Proceedings of the 3rd International Symposium of Circumpolar Health, Yellowknife, NWT, 8–11 July 1974. Toronto: University of Toronto Press. xv–xviii .

SISSONS, J. 1968. Judge of the Far North: The memoirs of Jack Sissons. Toronto: McClelland and Stewart Ltd.

STRUZIK, E. 1991. Northwest Passage: The quest of an Arctic route to the East. Toronto: Key Porter Books.

TODD, J. 1982. Doctor for a diseased civilization. *News/North*, June 25:A5.

VLESSIDES, M. 1997. Kekerten Historic Park. In: The 1998 Nunavut Handbook: Travelling in Canada's Arctic. Iqaluit: Nortext Multimedia Inc. 300–302.

Index

Page numbers appearing in italic type refer to pages that contain photographs. The abbreviation OS is used to indicate references to Otto Schaefer.

A

Adams, Willie, 208
adaptation to cold: International Biology Program research, 157–61, *158*; Inuit ways, 80, 198; Jack Hildes, 197–98; research by Vladimir Kaznacheyev, 178; traditional ways, 85
Adelaide Peninsula, 144–45, 191
Ahmi (Pangnirtung), 84–86
ai (right), 1
Aiyaoot (Spence Bay), 150–56, *151*
Aklavik, 15, 22, 23–26, *25, 26, 27,* 53, 148
Akshayuk (stepfather of Etuangat), *107,* 107–8
Alaska Highway, 135–36, 199
Alberta Achievement Award, 216
Alberta Hospital (Edmonton), 152
Alberta Medical Foundation, xi
Albrecht, C. Earl, 173, *177*
alcohol abuse: conference reports on, 175, 183; foetal alcohol syndrome, 136, 219; incidence, 136, 166, 169, 170; Iqaluit, 163; metabolism, 160, 219; Northern Medical Research Unit survey, 163, 166; social consequences, 135–37, 171, 183–84
Alikut, Guy, 172

All Saints Hospital (Aklavik), 24, 49
Allen, Bertha, 182
Amah (son of Kolitalik), 89–90
amauti (baby pouch), *94, 183,* 213, *214*
Amerongen, Betty, xi, 206
Amerongen, Gerald, xi, 113, 221
Amosie, wife of (son of Etuangat), *94*
Amosie (son of Etuangat), *5,* 80, 101, 117, *118, 119,* 164
Amundsen, Roald, 145
anaemia, 148, 179–80
Anchorage, Alaska, 173
Anerodluk, Paulette, 60, 72
angakok (shaman), 48–49, 81, 87–88, 110
Anglican Missions: Aklavik, 24, 49–50; early history, 17; Hay River, 48–49; Lake Harbour, 63; *Messenger,* 36; Pangnirtung, 75, 95, *99, 109,* 109–12, 110, *111;* support by OS, 111
antiseptic use of spruce gum, 29–30
archeology (Thule site, Pangnirtung), 112–14
Arctic Bay, 68, 158–59, 169
Arctic Red River, 21, 31–33, *33,* 35, 45–47, *46*
arctic willow *(Salix arctica),* 124
art and artists, Inuit: Baker Lake, *70;* Cape Dorset, 63; caribou carvings,

214; Ekootak (Holman Island), 183–84; Inukjuak, *65, 214, 216*; printmaking, 214; soapstone carvings and carvers, *65, 70*, 213–14, *214, 216*; Sugluk Inlet, 63; weavers, 187, 202
Arviat (Eskimo Point), *92,* 115–16, *129,* 147
Ashevaq (Illongaya), 88–89, *89*
Attuat (Arctic Bay), *69,* 183
auk (left), 1
aurora borealis, 91–92, *92*
Auyalo (Pangnirtung), 84–86
Auyuittuq National Park, 73, 74, *188,* 188–89, 212
Awtaktuk, 117
Ayaya (general approval), 93
Ayunamat (it can't be helped), 81

B

Back River, 144
Baden-Baden, Germany, 11
Baffin, William, 3–4, 62–63, 69
Baffin Island, 62–66
Baffin-Land, 7
Baillie Island, 41
Baker Lake, *70,* 147
Banks Island, 25
Banting, Frederick, 17
Barr, Cpl. (RCMP, Pangnirtung), 112–13
Bathurst Inlet, 49, *146*
Battle of the Bulge, 10
B.C. College of Physicians and Surgeons, 128
Beare, Maurice, xi, 81, 200–202, 219
Beare, Renata, xi
Beaufort Sea, 20, 36, 199
Berger Commission, 199
Betzdorf, Germany, 8, 10, 57
Billy (son of Rosie), 98
Binamé, Father, 36, 45–47, *46,* 49, 51

Black, Lyell, xi, 200
Boas, Franz, 54; as anthropologist, 7–8, 72, 111; influence on OS, 7–8, 67, 197, 203; view of Inuit, 16, 83, 217–18
Bonn, Germany, 8, 9
Boon, David and Joan, xi
breast-feeding, Inuit: advocacy by Jack Hildes, 198; advocacy by OS, 179–81, 182–84, 192, 197; benefits, 170, 179–81; bottle-feeding, 170, 179, *214*; as contraceptive, 180, 182, 192, 213–14, *214*; Inuit attitude toward, 108, *180*
Brett, Brian, vii–viii
Butler, Gordon, 147, 172, 181
Button, Thomas, 62–63
Bylot, Robert, 68–69
Bylot Island, 68, *68,* 184

C

Caesarean birth, 98–99
Canadian Armed Forces, 25, 112
Canadian Broadcasting Company, 53
Canadian Parks and Wilderness Society, 204–5
Canadian Physicians for the Prevention of Nuclear War, 179
Canadian Public Health Association, 221
Canadian Royal College, 127
Cape Dorset, 63, *65,* 129, *180,* 214
Cape Dyer, 84
capital punishment, 34–35
Cardinal, Mary Rose, 31–35
Cardinal, Sp. Const. Fred (RCMP, Arctic Red River), 31–35
caribou, 104, 115–16, 158, 163, 214
Castlegar, B.C., 128
Catholic Missions. *See* Roman Catholic Missions

C.D. Howe, 56, *58, 59, 67, 68,* 69, 148, *180, 213*; Baffin Island trips, vii, 62–73, 125; C. D. Howe, *59*; icebreaking, 59, 62
Central Arctic Surveys, 138, 144–49, 162
The Central Eskimo, 7–8, 197
Charles Camsell Hospital, 12, 14, 15, *16,* 18, 19, 37, 81, 127, 138–39, 152, 184, 185, 219
Chicksi, Millie, 19, *20*
childbirth, Inuit: death rates, 192; placenta, retained, 88–89, 148, 196; soapstone carving, *70*; traditional ways, 69–71, 81, 88–89
Chrétien, Jean, 176
Christensen, Axel, 22–25, *24*, 54, 97
Churchill Health Conference, *131*
Circumpolar Medical Conferences, 173–78, 190, 198
clothing and adornment, Inuit: *amauti* (baby pouch), *94, 183,* 213; hair, 27; *kamiks* (boots), 1, 118–19, *120*; parkas, 22; tattoos, *69*
Clyde River, *67*
Collins, Fred, 136
community health programs, 175–76, 198, 220
contraception, 180, 182, 192
Copenhagen, Denmark, 190
Coppermine, 60, 138, 146, *146,* 162–68, *164*
Coral Harbour, 66
Craig Harbour, *64*
Cree Indians, *16*
Crombie, David, 200, 202–3
Crozier, Capt. Frances, 144
Cumberland Sound, *5,* 74, *100, 116,* 121, 165

D

dance, drum, *92*, 92–93, 176

Davis, John, 74
Davis Strait, *56,* 63, 74
DC3, 83–84
demographics: acculturation, 191–92; Aklavik, 24; death and birth rates, 169, 191–92; frozen lung, 159; meningitis, 147; Northwest Territories, 143; Pangnirtung, 74–75, 165; Siberia, 175; suicide, 172; tuberculosis, 15, 63, 68, 192; unwed mothers, 170
dental care, Inuit, 39, 145–46, 166, *167,* 169; traditional ways, 88, *88,* 113, 119
Department of Health and Welfare, 17, 58, 130, 134, 136, 138–39, 147, 172, 200
Department of Indian and Eskimo Health Services, 12, 17, 139–40
Department of Indian and Northern Affairs, 142, 182, 184, 199
Devon Island, 71
DEW (Distant Early Warning) line, 53, 66, 111, 142, 163, 165
diabetes, 148, 160, 168
diarrhea, infant, 170, 179, 181
D'Iberville, 59, 71, *71*
Dier, Kay, xi, 127, 221
Digges Island, 69
Discovery, 64, 69
"diseases of civilization," 169–70
Doctor of Science Honorary Award, 217
Dogrib Indians, 176
dogs and dog teams: dog bites, *24,* 101; frozen lung research, 160; in Inuit myth, 215; life with, 42–43, 79–80, 119; medical transportation, 1–6, 75, 84–86, 100–104, *104,* 165, *188*; use in emergencies, 51, 105–7. See also *komatiks* (sleds)
Donaghue, Nancy, 134

Donaghue, Shirley, xi
drum dance, *92*
Drybones, Denise, 195

E

Eastern Arctic Patrol, vii, 57. See also *C.D. Howe*
Eastern Arctic Surveys, 145–49, 162
Edmonton, 200
Edwards, Allan M. ("Buzz"), xi, 127–28, 162, 207, 221–22
Ekootak (Holman Island), 183–84
elders, Inuit. *See* Attuat; Etuangat Aksayook
Ellesmere Island, 71, 129
epidemics: famine, 84, *115,* 115–16, 121–22; infant diarrhea, 181; influenza, 17; measles, 17, 146, 169; meningitis, 147; resistance to, 160; rubella (German measles), 97; smallpox, 169; suicide, 172; trichinosis, 119; tuberculosis, 63, 169; typhoid, 141; virus, 37; whooping cough, 17
Erebus, 144
Eskimo (eaters of raw meat), x, 82
"Eskimo lung," *159,* 159–60, 192
Eskimo Point (Arviat), *92*
Etuangat Aksayook: as assistant to OS, 1–4, *5,* 79–82, 100–104, 116–18, *188,* 210–11; as assistant to Schaefers, *76, 102*; Christmas in Pangnirtung, 94–95; as elder, 79–82, *80,* 112, 121–22, 208–11; hunting and fishing, *118*; Joapie (son), 79–80; Nukinga (wife), 81, *94,* 98, 164, 187; Order of Canada, 208–9, *209*; Paulusie (husband of Rosie), *97,* 117, 164, 187; reunions with OS, 164–65, 187, *210*. *See also* Rosie (Pangnirtung)
evacuation, medical: advocacy for, 17; destinations, 15–16, 58–59, 63, 86, 125; social consequences, 16, 42, 89, *129,* 130

F

famine, 84, *115,* 115–16, 121–22
fata morgana (mirages), 68
Feldscher community health program, 175
Fifth Thule Expedition of 1921–24, 190
food and nutrition, Inuit: breast-feeding, 179–81; impact of acculturation, 129–30, 148–49, 165–72, 179–81; infant iron supplements, 180–81; malnutrition, 168; sugar consumption, 166, 170; traditional diet, 104, 118–20, 180, 196
Forsius, Henrik, 177
Forsius, Mrs. Henrik, 177
Fort Churchill, 64
Fort Good Hope, 45–47
Fort Norman, 17
Fort Providence, 17
Fort Rae, 176, 195
Fort Resolution, 35
Fort Ross, 150–56
Fort Simpson, 20
Fort Smith, 35
Franklin Expedition, 57, 144–45, 191
Frobisher, Martin, 8, 66
Frobisher Bay (Iqaluit), 162–68
frostbite, 84–86, *85,* 108
frozen lung, *159,* 159–60, 192

G

Germania, 7
Gilbert, Allan, 128
Gjoa, 145
Gjoa Haven, 144, 145

Goodsoil, Saskatchewan, 12
Grainge, Jack, xi, 44
Great Fish (Back) River, 144
Great Slave Lake, 20, 35
Greenidge, Dr., 52–53
Grise Fiord, 57, 71
Groenlaendische Sagen (Tales of Greenland), 7, 191
Gruben, Charlie, 36–37
Guyasie (son of Paulusie), *97*

H

Hall Beach, 157–58
Hamilton, Ontario, 58
hardening of the arteries, 168
Hare Indians, 26, *26*
harpoons, 117–18, 215, *216*
health care, Indian: alcohol abuse, 135–37, 160, 219; birth rates, 169; Charles Camsell Hospital, 15; Cree Indians, *16*; Hare Indians, 26; Loucheux Indians, 24–26, 29–30, 39; Native Women's Conference, 182–84; research by OS, 134, 160; resistance to disease, 160; traditional ways, 29–30, 87
health care, Inuit: alcohol abuse, 160, 219; birth rates, 169; blood transfusions, 4–6; diabetes, 148, 160, 167; "diseases of civilization," 169–70; ear infections, 166, 170; frostbite, 84–86; frozen lung, 159–60, 192; gall bladder disease, 170; hardening of the arteries, 168; high blood pressure, 169; impact of acculturation, 144–49, 162–68, 169–72; infection, 41; lung cancer, 170; meningitis, 67, 147–48; mental illness, 2, 84, 151–56; Native Women's Conference, 182–84; pain tolerance, 127; resistance to disease, 160; women's

health care: lung cancer, 170. *See also* alcohol abuse; breastfeeding, Inuit; Charles Camsell Hospital; childbirth, Inuit; dental care, Inuit; evacuation, medical; tuberculosis
Heidelberg, University of, 10, 11
Heidi Schaefer Wilderness Preservation Award, 205
Hemophilus influenzae, 147–48
high blood pressure, 169
Hildes, Jack: archives, 193; collaboration with OS, 130–32, 138–39, 147, 157–61, 197–98, 213; conferences, *131,* 174–75; death, 198; friendship with OS, 132, 162, 198; Jack Hildes Medal, 217; research on adaptation to cold, 132, 157–61, *158,* 197–98
Hitler Youth, 9
Hoare Bay, 110, 147
Hodgson, Stuart M., 174
Holman Island, 138, 162–68, *163, 167*
homes, Inuit: humidification, 39, 148; igloo, *102,* 103–4, 158–59; tent/wooden hut, *97*; *tupik* (sealskin tent), 4, 103, 158–59
Houston, James, 63, 214
Howe, C. D., 59
Hudson, Henry, 64
Hudson Bay, 63
Hudson's Bay Company S. S. *Rupertsland,* 77
Hudson's Bay Company stores, *27,* 63, 74, 109, 163
hunting and fishing, Inuit: Baffin Island, 165; frozen lung, 159–60, 192; Hudson Bay, 69; muskrats, 24, 44–45; Pangnirtung, 115–22; polar bears, 119; respect for nature, 120; seals, 69, 118–19, *119*; tools, 116–17; walrus, 119; whales, 37, *45,* 116–18, *118*

I

iceberg, *56*
icebreakers, 59, 62, *71*. See also *C.D. Howe*
igloo, 85, *102*, 103–4
Igloolik, 89, 157–58, *158*, *159*
Ihalmiut (Kazan River), *92*
Illongaya, 1–2, *5*, 6, *89*
Immaculate Conception Hospital (Aklavik), 24, 36, 49
Indian Friendship Society (Whitehorse), 137
Indian health care. *See* health care, Indian
Indians. *See* Hare Indians; Loucheux Indians
infanticide, female, 191
INH (Isonicotinic Acid Hydrazide), 220
International Biology Program research, 157–61
International Congress of Nutrition (Prague), 179
International Polar Year, First, 7, 203
International Whaling Commission, 116
Inugsuin Fiord, *67*
Inuit. *See also* art and artists, Inuit; childbirth, Inuit; clothing and adornment, Inuit; dental care, Inuit; food and nutrition, Inuit; health care, Inuit; homes, Inuit; hunting and fishing, Inuit; justice, Inuit and NWT system of; tuberculosis
Inuit languages, 26, 66. *See also* Inuktitut
Inuit physical features, 26–27, 66, 158, *158*
Inuit (the People), x, 82
Inuk (an individual), 82
Inukjuak (Port Harrison), 65, 213–14, *214*

Inuktitut: Boas, 7; dialects, 66; and English, 26, 142; Etuangat as teacher, 3, 81–82; names, 108; Pangnirtung, 81; proverb on good wives, 202; syllabics, 84, 142, 154
Inusilk (Shaunitoratiuk), 103
Inuvik, 53, 158–59, 169
Iqaluit (Frobisher Bay), 162–68, *167*
iron, supplemental, 180–81
Iruk, Selena, 213
Itlaut, 184
Ivuyivik, 63

J

Jacobsen, Mike, 41
Jacobsen, Vera, 41, *41*
Joanasie (Pangnirtung), *110*
Joapie (son of Etuangat), 79–80
Johnson, Albert, 23–24
Johnson's Crossing, 135
Josie (husband of Soosee), 171–72
justice, Inuit and NWT system of: assisted suicide of Kolitilik, 89–90; murder of Soosee, 150–56

K

Kadloo (father of Shooyook), 150, 154
kadluna (white foreigners), 79–80, 156
kamiks (boots), 1, 118–19, *120*
kayaks (boats), 116, *116*
Kazan River drummer, *92*
Kaznacheyev, Vladimir Ilyich Lenin ("Vlail"), *177*, 177–78, 190, 213
Keewatin District, *115*, 145, 147, 190–91
Kekerten Island, 165
killaluga (beluga or white whale), 116–18
King William Island, 144, 191
Kingnait Fiord, *104*, 112–14
Kittigazuit, 37, *38*

Knud Rasmussen Memorial Lecture, 190–91
Kolitalik (Igloolik), 89–90
Komaiki, Const. P.E. (RCMP, Arctic Red River), 31–32
komatiks (sleds), 1–6, *5,* 79, 84–86, 100–104, *101*
Koviachukbi (May you be happy), 95

L

Labrador Stream, 62
Lake Harbour (Kimmirut), 62–63
lamps, seal-oil, 103, 104, 118, 213
Lancaster Sound, 63, 69, *71*
The Land of the Long Day, 184
languages, Arctic, 26. *See also* Inuktitut
Larson, Insp. (RCMP, Pangnirtung), 113
Laurent-Christensen, Axel. *See* Christensen, Axel
Learmonth, L.A., 155
LeBlanc, Gov. Gen. Roméo, 208, *209*
legends and myths, Inuit: aurora borealis, 92; dogs, 215; Fr. M. Metayer, 176; storyteller, 48–49
Léger, Gov. Gen. Jules, 200, *201*
Levesque, Fr. Gilbert, 32–33
Licentiate of the Medical Council of Canada (LMCC), 14
Livingstone, Leslie, 17, 75–76, 82
Loucheux Indians, *27*; Arctic Red River, 31; Fred Cardinal case, 31–35; languages, 26; Lazarus Sittichiulis, 24; "Mad Trapper" case, 23–24; muskrat trade, 24; Old Crow, 39, 182; Rev. James Sittichinli, 49–50, *50*
Lougheed, Peter, 216
lung cancer, 170
Luttakulu (dear little doctor), 22, 222
Luttamiut (doctor's people), *94*

M

Mackenzie, Alexander, 20
Mackenzie Delta, 21, *21,* 37
Mackenzie Mountain Range, 21
Mackenzie River, 20, 25, *27, 28,* 28–29, 199
MacNeish, R.S., 37, 113
MacPherson, A.D., 154
"Mad Trapper of Rat River," 23–24
Makpa (Baker Lake), *70*
malnutrition, 168
Marsh, Rev. Donald, *111*
Martin, J. D., 193
McBride, Boyd, 34
McCallum, Arnold, 193
McCarten, Alan, 206
McGill University, 181
McLaughlin, Sgt. (RCMP, Aklavik), 31–34
measles, 146, 169
Melville Peninsula, 89
meningitis, 67, 147–48
mental illness, 2, 84, 151–56
Merrill, Curt, 53
Messenger, 36
metabolism, 160
Metayer, Fr. M., 176
missionaries, 48–51, 111–12, 162. *See also* Anglican Missions; Roman Catholic Missions
Moffet Inlet, 112
Montreal Arts Guild, 63
Morrow, William, 154
Mosesie (Inukjuak), *65, 216*
Mowat, Farley, 155–56
muktuk (whale skin), 104
music, *92,* 92–93, 142, 176
muskrats, 24, 44
Mussell, Bill, 176

N

Namao Air Force base, 184
Napachee-Kadlac (husband of Soosee), 153, 154
Napoleon (Inuit hunter, Aklavik), 27–28
narwhal, *118,* 215
National Film Board of Canada, 184
National Museum, 37, 113
Native Women's Conference, 182–84
Naudla (Cumberland Sound), *101*
Nemetz, Emmi, xi, 127, 135
Norman Wells, 21
Norseman, 19–22, *20,* 52, 145
North Battleford, Saskatchewan, 13
Northern Medical Research Unit: establishment of, 139–40; Holman Island laboratory, *163;* research, 144–49, 162–72
Northern Science Award Centenary Medal, *202*
Northwest Passage, search for, 57, 62–63
Northwest Territories, 17
Northwest Territories Justice Department, 31–35, 89, 150–56
Northwest Territories Water Board, 195, 199
Novosibirsk, Siberia, 177, 178, 190
Nukinga (wife of Etuangat), 81, *94,* 98, 164, 187

O

obesity, 169
Old Crow, 25, 39, *40,* 133, 182
Order of Canada, 200
Order of Grey Nuns, 17
Osborne, Jim, 81
Otoki (Cape Dorset), *88*
Ottawa, 200–203, 208–9
Otto Schaefer Health Resource Centre, 193–94, *194*
Oulu, Finland, 173, 177

P

Padlermiut, *115*
Padloping, 72
Paege, Winnie, xi
pan-abode house, 165
Pangnirtung: Anglican Mission, *109,* 109–12, *111;* art centre, 187; Christmas, *93,* 93–95, *94;* climate, 91; community life, 73–78, *75;* Livingstone, Leslie, 17, 75–76, 82; Native Women's Conference, 182–84; Northern Medical Research Unit, 162–68; as paradise, x, 74, 78, 125–26, 164–65, 185, 187–89, 215, 217; Schaefer home, 76, *76,* 96, 107, *107,* 120–21; Schaefers, *77, 123, 218;* waterfalls, *124;* whaling, 116–18
Pangnirtung Fiord, *72,* 74, *75, 118,* 217
Parker, John H., 193, 195
Paulusie (husband of Rosie), *97,* 117, 164, 187
Peace River, 20
Peel Channel, *28*
Peel River, 29
Pelly Bay, 145, *183*
Penny, William, 165
Penny Ice Cap, 72–73, 189
Pililuk, Kenneth and Sarah, 44, *45*
pneumonia, 97, 99, 147
Point Separation, 46
Pokiak, Maurice, *38*
polar bears, 119, 134–35, 158, 215
Pond Inlet, *60,* 68, *68*
Prickett, Abacuck, 64
Procter, Harry, 138–40
Pungnana, Lena, *24*

R

Raddy, Sam, 136
Rae River, 146
Rankin Inlet, 147, 208
Rasmussen, Knud, 7, 190–91
RCMP, 109, 112–13, 150, 152–55
religious beliefs: *angakok* (shaman), 48–49, 81; animals, 120; Pangnirtung, 110; religious leaders, 48–51, 111; spells and curses, 153. *See also* Anglican Missions; Roman Catholic Missions
Resolute Bay, *58, 60,* 69, 184, 215
Resolution Island, 67
Reubsatt, Helmut, 128
Richardson Mountains, *21*
rickets, 98, 166
rifles, 117–18, 153, 175
Roberts, Vera, 98–99, *99,* 105–7, 110, 200, *202,* 211
Robinson, Dorothy ("Robbie"), *99,* 113
Roman Catholic Missions, 17, *33, 35, 46,* 49
Ronald, A. R., 147
Rosie (Pangnirtung), *94,* 94–95, *97,* 98–99, 164
Rossall, Dick, xi, 128
Royal Alexandra Hospital, *13,* 13–14
Royal Canadian Air Force, *93, 93*
rubella, 97

S

Saami, 175
Sabean, B., 81
Sabine, Dr., 125
Salluit, 214
Salter, Madeleine, 98
Samonie, *120*
Schaefer, Alfred (Otto and Didi's son), 57, *59, 77, 94,* 120, 212

Schaefer, Editha (Didi)
EARLY LIFE: medical assistant in Pang, 98–99
FAMILY AND PERSONAL LIFE: birth of Lothar, 54; birth of Taoya, 82; Canadian citizenship, 128; conservationist, 199, 205; courtship and marriage, 4, *14,* 14–15; death, 206–7; death of Heidi, 204–5; early career, 14–15; Edmonton home, 200, 212–18; health, 105–7, *106,* 124–25, 205–7; language skills, 15, 81; later travels with family, 187–89, 193–94, 200–203, *206, 207*; love of outdoors, 54, 123–26, 185, 188–89, 207; relationship with Otto, 15, 139–40, 185–89, 205–7
LIFE IN THE ARCTIC: in Aklavik, 19–22, *20,* 25, 44–47, *45, 54,* 54–55; on *C.D. Howe,* 57, *59,* 72–73; in Pangnirtung, 74–78, *77,* 92–95, 98–99, 105–8, *106,* 117, 120–21, *121,* 123–26; Pangnirtung as paradise, 74, 78, 125–26, 164–65, 185, 187–89, 215, 217; personal writing, 46–47, 54, 74; visit to Old Crow, 39, *40,* 133; in Whitehorse, 133–34
Schaefer, Heidi (Otto and Didi's daughter), 204–5, *205,* 212
Schaefer, Joseph (Otto's brother), 7–8
Schaefer, Lizbeth (Otto's sister), 8
Schaefer, Lothar (Otto and Didi's son), *54, 59,* 59–60, *77,* 120, 186, 207, 212
Schaefer, Monika (Otto and Didi's daughter), 185, 204, 212
Schaefer, Otto (OS)
ADVOCATE FOR ARCTIC PEOPLE: against alcohol abuse, 135–37, 183–84, 219; for breastfeeding, 179–81, 183;

248 • Index

for community health programs, 220; for good nutrition, 162–68, 172, 183; for missionaries, 111; for preserving historical sites, 112–14; tenacity in advocacy, 172. See also Hildes, Jack

AWARDS AND HONOURS: Alberta Achievement Award, 216; Commissioner's Award for Public Service at the Highest Level (Yellowknife), 193; Doctor of Science Honorary Award, 217; Jack Hildes Medal, 217; Knud Rasmussen Memorial Lecture, 190–92; Northern Science Award Centenary Medal, *202*, 202–3; Order of Canada, 200, *201*; Ortho Award, 221

EARLY CAREER (Edmonton, Aklavik, Pangnirtung, Whitehorse): in Aklavik, 18–47, *40*, 52–55; Canadian citizenship, 128; Canadian medical exams, 12–14, 127, 128; on *C.D. Howe*, 56–73; Edmonton hospitals, viii, *13*, 13–18, 97, 127–28, 198; in Pangnirtung, 1–6, 74–126, *100*; trial of Fred Cardinal, 31–35; in Whitehorse, 133–37. See also Etuangat Aksayook

EARLY INFLUENCES ON OS: Arctic dreams, 7–8, 11, 57, 62–66; Boas, Franz, 7–8, 54; immigration to Canada, 3, 12–13; life in Germany, 3, 7–11, 128; Rasmussen, Knud, 7, 190–191

FAMILY AND SOCIAL LIFE: in Aklavik, *54*; on *C.D. Howe*, *59*; celebrations, 39–40, 72, 92–95, 187, 193–95, 200–203; deaths, 204–7, 211; Edmonton home, 212–18; as father, 186–87, 212; life with Didi, *14*, 14–15, 19, 36, 44–47, 92–95, 139–40, 185–89, 205–7, 217; Pangnirtung, *106*, *123*, *210*; Pangnirtung as paradise, 78, 125–26, 185, 187–89, 217–18, *218*. See also Etuangat Aksayook; Schaefer, Editha (Didi)

LATER CAREER (Northern Medical Research Unit and after): Berger Commission, 199; Churchill Health Conference, *131*; Circumpolar Medical Conferences, 173–78, *174*, *177*, 190, 198; Dr. Otto Schaefer Health Resource Centre, 193, *194*; Edmonton hospitals, 138–40; International Congress of Nutrition, 179; Knud Rasmussen Memorial Lecture, 190–92; Native Women's Conference, 182–84; Northern Medical Research Unit, 138–49, 162–68, *163*, *164*; Water Board of the Northwest Territories, 199; witness in Soosee trial, 150–56

PERSONAL LIFE: attitude to food, 44, 104, *104*, 132, 162; eagerness to learn, 9, 98, 128, 186, 196; frugality, 104, 199; interest in anthropology, 58, 112–14; language skills, 3, 8, 15, 18, 26, 81, 128, 216; modesty, 176; nickname *shik-shik*, 22, 37, 217; outdoors life (skiing in Edmonton), 162; physical features and health, 3, 6, 9, 18, 52–53; temperament, 9, 127, 172, 186, 221; writing habits, 6, 129, 196

RESEARCH AND PUBLICATIONS: collaboration with Jack Hildes, 157–61; diet and nutrition research, 162–68; evaluation of his contributions, 219–22; notebooks, 37–38, 70–71, 129, 196, 216, 221; Otto Schaefer Health Resource Centre, 193, *194*; publications, 196–98; research on human

adaptation to cold, 157–61, *158*; role of Jack Hildes, 130–32, 197–98; theories, 127; view of women's role in health care, 182
Schaefer, Taoya. *See* White, Taoya
schizophrenia, Inuit response to, 150–56
Schneider, Bill, 12–13
seals, 118–19, *119*
Searle, David, 150
shaman *(angakok)*, 48–49, 81, 87–88, 110
Shaunitoratiuk (place of many bones), 103
shik-shik (Arctic ground squirrel) as OS nickname, 22, 37, 217
Shooyook (Spence Bay), 150–56, *151*
Siberia, 175
Siedbach, Richard, 10, 11
Simionie (Inukjuak), *214*
Sissons, Judge John (Jack), 89, 150, *153,* 155–56, 185
Sittichinli, Rev. James, 49–50, *50*
Sittichiulis, Lazarus, 24, *26*
Skilak, 176
sled, Inuit. See *komatiks* (sled)
smallpox, 169
Smith, Cameron, 155
smoking, 170
Smythe, Rev. and Mrs., 111
snowmobiles, 75, 165, 175, 200
social behaviour, Inuit: acculturation, 141–43, 169–72, 182–84; *ayunamat* (it can't be helped), 81; celebrations, 94–95, 176; family life, 176; hardships, 83–86; impact of acculturation on families, 170–72; interdependence, 121–22, 160–61; names, Inuit, 108; need for acceptance, 171–72; preserving community, 154–55; stoicism, 27–28, 84–86, 127; suicide, 89–90, 183–84; supernatural beliefs, 153, 154; training, 79–80, 122, 214; women's roles, 119, 142. *See also* childbirth, Inuit; Etuangat Aksayook; hunting and fishing, Inuit; justice, Inuit and NWT system of
Soosee (Spence Bay), 150–56, *152, 171*
Southampton Island, 66
Spence Bay, 138, 150–56, *151,* 184
spring breakup, 25, *28,* 28–29, 75
spruce gum as antiseptic, 29–30
S.S. *Arctic,* 75
S.S. *Atlantic,* 12
S.S. *Rupertsland,* 77, 94–95
St. Luke's Hospital (Pangnirtung), 75, *99, 109*
Stalin, 178
Stanton Hospital (Yellowknife), 193
Starvation Cove, 191
storytelling, Inuit, 48–49
Stout, Iris, xi, 134, 135, 185
sugar consumption, 166
Sugluk (Salluit) Inlet, 63
suicide, 89–90, 171–72, 175, 183–84
Summit Lake, *187, 188,* 188–89, *206,* 212
Sunchild Cree, *16*
Sunshine, 74
Supik (Craig Harbour), *64*
sweating, Inuit, 158, *158*

T

Tabawutit (good-bye), 125, 211
Tapitia (Cape Dyer), 84, 116
tattoos, Inuit, *69*
Taylor, Elva, xi, 18, 185, 205
Terror, 144
Teslin Lake, 135
Third International Symposium on Circumpolar Health. *See* Circumpolar Medical Conferences

Thule site (Pangnirtung), 112–14
Tinling, Shorty, 105, 109
trials: assisted suicide of Kolitilik, 89–90; murder of Marie Cardinal, 31–35; murder of Soosee, 150–56
trichinosis, 119, 134–35
Trudeau, Pierre, 69
tuberculosis: community health programs, 138, 175; death rates, 148, 169, 192; evacuation, 89, 129–30; hospitals, 58, *109*; incidence, 15–16, 24, 63, 68, 130, 148, 166, 175; INH (Isonicotinic Acid Hydrazide), 220; meningitis, 67, 147; resistance to, 68, 160
Tuktoyaktuk, 36–37, *38, 45*
tupik (sealskin tent), 4, 103
Turner, Arthur, 164
Turner, Rev. John, 81, 98, 112, 184
Twapait, *100*
typhoid, *100*, 141

U

umiaks (boats), 116
Ungava Bay, 62, 66
University Hospital (Edmonton), 15, 127, 198
University of Manitoba, 130, 131, 147, 217
Utaluk (Pangnirtung), *110*

V

vaccines, *100,* 146, 148
vegetation, Arctic, 19, 21, 36, 77, 120, 123–24
Veitch, Joe, 41–43, *42,* 54
venereal disease, 169, 170, 175
Victoria Strait, 144
Victory Point, 144
Vitali, Wilfred, 189

W

Walker Bay, *167*
Wallator, Ken, 204
walrus, 119
walrus carving, *216*
walrus dentures, *88*
Webster, Ann, 60–61
Webster, Rev. J. Harold, 49–51, 60, 101, 145
Wehrmacht (German army), 9–10
Westgate, Norma, xi, 37, 39, 77–78, 96, *99,* 110
whales and whaling, 66, 102, 116–18, *118,* 214, 215
White, Taoya (Otto and Didi's daughter), xi, 82, 108, 179, 185, 199–200, 208, 212
Whitefish Station, *45*
Whitehorse, 134
Whyard, Flo, 137
Williams, Gwen, *99*
Williams, Tom, 206
Wingek, Cyril, 48–49, *49*
women, Inuit: Native Woman's Conference, 182–84; proverb, 103, 202; tuberculosis rates, 130, 192. *See also* breast-feeding; childbirth, Inuit

Y

Yellowknife, 19–20, 34–35, 173–75, 193–95, *194*
Yonge, Keith A., 154
Yukon Territories, 133–34

Z

Zubko, Mike, 39, 40, 52